This Works Crutches Don't

Why Healing Your Bowel Will Eliminate Your Symptoms, Illness, Addictions, and Weight Struggles and Why Crutches—Diets, Vitamins, Drugs, Exercise, etc.—Don't

Donna Pessin, Certified Nutritional Consultant
www.ThisWorksCrutchesDont.com

authorHOUSE®

AuthorHouse™
1663 Liberty Drive, Suite 200
Bloomington, IN 47403
www.authorhouse.com
Phone: 1-800-839-8640

First published by AuthorHouse   4/27/2009

ISBN: 978-1-4389-4281-0 (sc)

Printed in the United States of America
Bloomington, Indiana

This book is printed on acid-free paper.

Warning/Disclaimer

This book is designed to provide information on healing your bowel and body, and eliminating symptoms, illness, future disease, addictions, and weight struggles. The purpose of this book is to educate and inspire. It is sold with the understanding that the author is not a medical professional and that this advice has not been proven scientifically. The information in this book is not intended to diagnose or treat disease, or to replace the recommendations of your medical doctor. The reader must understand that it is their constitutional right to decide how they wish to care for the health of their body. The author has not suggested that the reader cease current medical care, be it drug therapy, x-ray treatment, chemotherapy, surgery, or any other medical procedures that their medical doctor deems necessary to their health. If the reader chooses to not follow recommendations made by their medical doctor, they understand that such a decision is their responsibility and will not hold the author responsible for any consequences of such a decision. The author shall have neither liability nor responsibility to any person or entity with respect to any damage caused, or alleged to have been caused, directly or indirectly, by the information contained in this book. Every effort has been made to make this book as complete and accurate as possible. However, there may be mistakes, both typographical and in content. Therefore, this book should be used only as a general guide and not as the ultimate source for healing your bowel and body. Furthermore, this book contains information on healing the bowel and body that is current only up to the printing date.

Healing your bowel and body is not a simple, quick fix, process. Anyone who decides to heal their bowel and body must expect to invest a lot of time and effort into it. For many people, this process has resulted in a complete elimination of their symptoms, illness, addictions, and weight problems.

Table of Contents

Introduction

My Story

The years prior to my devastating illness—alcoholism, drug use, eating disorder

At a young age, I became involved in drugs and alcohol. Initially, I used these because they allowed me to escape the anxiety and emptiness of living in a very dysfunctional home. My favorite drug was pot. I loved how it numbed me and helped me ignore the reality of my life. It made me feel calm and safe, and this was very appealing.

By the time I was sixteen, my reasons for drinking and doing drugs had changed. I could drink a lot more than before, and alcohol had become much more than an escape for me; it had become something I craved. The conscious decision to numb myself had turned into a need. I was having a hard time coping without my drugs. I was becoming dependent on them, not just emotionally, but physically as well.

I came home very drunk many nights, even during the school week. After only a few hours of sleep, however, I could get up, go to class, and get an "A." I thought I was getting away with it.

I started to experiment with other drugs too (and eventually used most of them). At this point I started blacking out. Ironically, this was a positive experience, because blacking out my reality was better than dealing with it. It was only years later, once I stopped drinking, that I realized the danger I had put myself in while driving home from bars on the winding roads of my home town of Chappaqua, NY, with no memory the next day of having done so.

By the time I got to college I was drinking excessively and blacking out all the time, but I continued to get "A's," and I continued to feel ok. In fact, I never got sick—not just from too much alcohol, but with the flu or a cold, either. I saw these as signs that I wasn't hurting myself with my abuses. Deep down, however, I had a very unstable, out of control feeling, which I continued to numb with more alcohol and drugs.

In high school and college I starved myself all day to keep my weight down. I understood that being thin got me more attention, and I constantly struggled and obsessed about my weight. By night, I was consuming large quantities of alcohol, which was often followed by a period of uncontrollable binging on sugary or starchy foods. The next day, upset with myself for having eaten that much the night before, I would starve myself again, with the pattern repeating itself over and over again. Often the only lunch I ate was a small salad, about the size of a deck of cards, or a bag of corn nuts. I counted calories obsessively. I knew that the alcohol added up to calories and because I could not stop drinking, I forced myself to stop eating.

The morning my life changed

When I was twenty-two years old, over twenty years ago, it all caught up with me. Overnight, I was faced with a devastating illness that left me completely disabled for many years, and fighting for my life. It completely and dramatically changed my health and life as I knew it.

After college I landed a job selling large corporate health insurance policies with Metropolitan Life Insurance Company. (I accepted this job after being offered one as a pharmaceutical sales rep in Beverly Hills for Pfizer, a fact I found quite ironic, given my current job and passion.) I was living in southern California, and the company sent me and several other new employees to Manhattan for a three-week sales training program. I drank heavily most nights. During the day I had to sit in what I found to be very boring training sessions, so showing up tired, incoherent, and very jittery was not a problem, except that I had never felt that way before. Something felt very different, a feeling I tried to erase by drinking more. At the time, of course, I was an alcoholic, but like many in those shoes, this never dawned on me.

Then one morning I woke up feeling extremely shaky. It was far worse than ever before. I had the sensation that my head and upper body were completely disconnected from my lower body. My brain was in a complete fog. These sensations did not go away. As the days went by and they continued I knew, deep inside, that my body was on its way out. The realization of this, along with having absolutely no knowledge of if or how I could reverse it, was the most frightening experience of my life. I quit drinking immediately.

As the weeks went by I experienced severe anxiety attacks; constant jittery, shaky feelings that left me completely unable to function. These lasted twenty-four hours a day and for many years. Driving was near impossible. I also had daily, crippling neck and chest pain, horrific insomnia and fatigue, an inability to concentrate, and severe hypoglycemia. Even though I had stopped drinking, I felt incoherent and unstable on my feet, as though I were drinking still. I had food allergies that landed me in the hospital and environmental allergies that practically caused me to "live in a bubble." I battled with depression, Candida, PMS, headaches, and constipation. These horrible symptoms plagued me for years.

Years of disability

Shortly after the episode in New York, I was forced to quit my job. I thought that when I stopped drinking I would be ok, but I never got better. I spent 2 ½ years on complete disability and I spent every day of this in total fear. I felt as though every second of the day I had to focus on compelling my body to stay alive.

During the first 1-½ years of my illness, I saw twenty-five medical doctors. Most of them were very disrespectful to me. Very few tests were done to determine what was wrong, although a prominent infectious disease specialist eventually gave me the vague label of having an autoimmune disease. At the time I became ill, AIDS, M.S., fibromyalgia, and even chronic fatigue syndrome were diseases that were widely unheard of and unknown in the medical field. If you presented yourself to a doctor with symptoms of one of these, you were usually told that it was "all in your head." I was told I would have to learn to live with my symptoms and I was given some drugs to try to decrease them. I knew deeply that more drugs, albeit pharmaceutical ones, would be the nails in my coffin and that this was not an acceptable answer. The answer, however, was something I didn't have.

I'm not jumping off the bridge

Living with my symptoms was not an option for me. I concluded that I had two choices at this point: jump off a bridge, or travel down a different road. Obviously I chose the later. I was given the name of an alternative medical doctor practicing experimental medicine in Newport Beach. I spent a number of months seeing him but received no benefit from his program. Later on he was sent to jail for his practices.

My second experience in alternative health was with a nutritionist who recommended dozens of supplements and a high protein, anti-Candida diet. His program was very much like the majority of programs offered by most alternative health practitioners today. After one year on this program, I was in an even deeper black hole, physically. My health and symptoms were worse than ever. I was hanging on by a thread. The next person I saw was a homeopath who thought I was dying from AIDS. I moved on from this man after many months of seeing minimal improvement.

Altogether I went to twenty or more alternative practitioners, including herbalists, chiropractors, acupuncturists, and massage therapists—all in search of a way to feel normal again. Only later on, when I was completely healthy, did I realize that my "normal" was actually very unhealthy.

Ten years searching for health

I spent ten years trying to regain my health and get my life back. I tried every anti-Candida diet on the market, along with all of the supplements that were recommended then, as they are today, to treat it. I even took an illegal drug from France when none of the others worked. I was put on food allergy diets, fasts, and given countless more herbs and supplements. I spent two years having all of my amalgam fillings removed. I spent four hours a week sitting in a doctor's office with an I.V. in my arm delivering oxygen and mega-nutrients, including very high levels of vitamin C, into my body. I had vitamin B-12 and gamma globulin shots in my behind. I did over 450 enemas and some 80 colonics. For seven months I ate nothing but millet, vegetables, and rice protein powder. I diligently followed dairy-free, wheat-free, enzyme-rich diets for years. I properly combined meals. I practiced visualization, affirmations, meditation, biofeedback, and deep breathing. I exercised frequently, as I had been doing when I first became very ill. **I took anything and practically everything that was recommended then, as it is today, to eliminate my symptoms.**

I was thoroughly and strictly committed to these programs, but none of them worked. I only began to see considerable changes when I decided to take the matter into my own hands and started to apply the principles in this book. When all else had failed, I decided to go back to school to continue my studies in nutrition. During all of the years that I had been sick, I had been reading about alternative health and attending as many health seminars as possible to learn how to heal my body. I spent thousands and thousands of hours trying to figure this all out.

What finally worked

Early on in my illness I read about the importance of bowel health, and when all else failed, I returned to this concept, which had always made sense to me. I learned how to heal my bowel and how to safely, but aggressively, eliminate the enormous storage of acids/ toxins in my body. This accomplished a permanent healing of my body that all of the other programs, which only treat the symptoms of an overly acidic body, never would or could accomplish. The information that I am presenting in this book is "what finally worked."

More importantly, the information in this book has continued to work for many years. Numerous programs offer short-term fixes that fail in the long run. This program delivers long-term results.

My results

My journey was very long and extremely painful, but it was by far the best thing I have experienced in my life. It gave me a life. Today I am the healthiest and happiest that I have ever been. I have no more neck or chest pain, no anxiety, no depression, no constipation, no hypoglycemia, no PMS, a lot of energy, no insomnia, and no difficulty maintaining my weight. I have not drunk alcohol in twenty years and abstaining from it is completely effortless. My eating disorder mentality is gone. Because I healed my body, I crave healthy foods, but I do not need to follow a strict diet or limit my carbohydrates to look and feel good. I tolerate high levels of wheat and dairy when once even the smallest amount left me crippled for days. I eat a low protein, high carbohydrate diet. I do not need extra supplements to maintain these results, either. **My healthy body—and not a diet, exercise, or a bunch of supplements—keeps my weight down and me feeling fabulous. My fear of becoming ill with cancer or any other disease, and of losing control of my weight, is completely gone. This outcome alone is priceless.**

My passion and dream

I am extremely passionate about, and committed to, helping others attain the unbelievable physical and mental health that I have. I have helped many clients achieve this even when all else has failed. I have helped many clients eliminate conditions that modern medicine calls incurable. I hope to sell millions of copies of this book, because the more people I can help, the better. On the largest scale, my dream is to help prevent as much suffering that I can. I suffered a great deal when I was younger and when I was ill. I know the pain, and I also know that much of it can be prevented and eliminated.

If I had to choose only three conditions to work with in my practice they would be infertility, addictions, and eating disorders. I had no problems getting pregnant myself, but infertility inspires me because I think this is the most powerful way to positively affect the health and weight of future generations. Addictions and eating disorders are a passion because of my personal experiences. These two conditions are very similar in many ways, and one day, I hope to open treatment centers that work with both.

And one day, I would like to give back to less-fortunate communities and individuals through a non-profit organization aimed at educating others how to heal their bodies. I have been given more than one can imagine, and I have much to give back.

Why Me?

I am often asked why it is that I have the knowledge to heal the body and others don't. Why do I have the answer when everyone else they have seen, including prestigious medical and alternative health practitioners, does not? When a client does not ask this question, I can often see it forming in their mind. Why me? I too have asked myself that question many times. Of course I cannot answer that question with anything but a guess, and some additional insight into how I got here.

Timing and location

I became ill at a time when the published books of great minds and healers were still on the shelves of the health food stores. Back then it wasn't all about treating symptoms with crutches, like it is now. I had easy and wide access to information that is much more difficult, and in some cases, impossible, to find now. I was also living in southern California at the time, where I had access to a very progressive alternative movement that would have been difficult to find elsewhere. Twenty years ago I was exposed to, and tried, therapies that many others are just today calling revolutionary.

I love to read

I could spend weeks curled up on a chair at the beach with a stack of good books and be perfectly content. When I was ill, I read a lot. I read books on health and nutrition all day long. I was disabled so I *had* all day long to read! Some of these books I read at least thirty times, desperately trying to figure out how to use the knowledge to heal myself. I have always been an "A" student and I learn easily. This self-taught knowledge turned out to be the most helpful to me in finding the answer to my health problems.

A little luck, a lot of experience, and hard work

Over sixteen years ago I began a private practice to help and teach others what I had learned. Luckily, I got on the "right road" early on in my practice. As a practitioner I was very alone on this road, but there was no way I was getting off of it. I have the extreme advantage of having years of experience applying what I knew with many clients and learning even more as I went along. I was in a position to test and perfect this approach. This work and book did not come easily. It is the product of thousands of hours of sacrifice and hard work.

No financial pressures or ego

Throughout this journey, I felt like the luckiest woman alive for all that I had been through and learned. I did not "need" success to feel worthy. I felt that I had received more than enough. My need to learn was far more important than my need for recognition. For example, when I first went back to school to study nutrition I was in a Masters of Science program working towards a M.S. degree and subsequent certification as a Dietician. I believed that the degree and certification would bring with it a degree of credibility and respect. One day as I was sitting in biochemistry class I looked at a letter I had just received in the mail advertising a certification program in alternative health. I reviewed the course descriptions and became very excited, much more excited than I had ever been about the curriculum I was currently studying. That was my "the apple hit my head" moment. I realized that I was never going to learn the depth of healing that I was looking for in the current program, and that helping people was much more important than having fancy credentials. I knew then and there that I had to change my course. My teachers were shocked—it was mid-trimester and I was an "A" student, for goodness sake. "A" students did not typically drop out of the program.

I was fortunate to have some financial support while I was searching for the answers to health and healing. This enabled me to find an unbiased approach to the answer and was critical to my getting where I am today. In this field there is great temptation to make money by selling the quick fix. A lot of money can be made off of supplement sales. I let go of those temptations and proceeded down this path with the sole intent of learning as much as I could to help others heal. The financial outcome was not the motivation. I have made less money than I would have had I gone down the more common road of treating symptoms with crutches. But by not going down that road, I was able to find this road of healing. *You can't be on both roads at the same time.*

Three keys to my success

I have worked with many clients who have struggled with weight and health problems, and while this program is the missing link, something none of them had ever tried prior to seeing me, there is something even more powerful than this program that you need to succeed. I have thought about this often. How did I ever find the answer to my problems and eventually transform my life? The three keys to my success were:

1. I never gave up.
2. I saw all of my failures as opportunities to learn.
3. I forgave myself for all of the wrongs I had done.

Was I chosen to do this?

Ultimately, I think the answer to this question is "yes." Who chose me? I don't know. I believe in a spiritual world, but I do not know who, exactly, chose me. I have had a lot of experiences in my life and can relate to many people in many different states of mental and physical health. Others relate to me as well, so I am a good "choice" for spreading this information.

Writing a book takes a lot of time and commitment. The energy needed to do this, as well as to deal with the consequences of writing it, are great, and many times I tried to ignore the need to write this book. Every time I did, something happened (it always seemed like an obvious sign), that got me back on track and made me realize that I needed to write this. *I waited for someone else to write "this book" and share this information, and when no one did, I realized that it was up to me to do so.*

More than anything, I simply have a deep down feeling that it is my responsibility to share this information with you. At the very least, I know that sharing this work is definitely my purpose in life.

This Book Is for You If…

You believe you can heal your body; if you believe that your body was not designed to feel bad and struggle with its weight; if you believe that there is an answer and that the answer involves a natural, alternative approach.

You understand that drugs are not the answer; that they simply treat your symptoms but mask the cause of your problems, and that they are not healthy for your body and you are rightly concerned about using them and/or becoming addicted to them.

You don't want to, and can't, take supplements or follow a strict diet the rest of your life, and think this shouldn't be necessary to maintain your health and weight anyway! If you are on a strict low carbohydrate or food-allergy program and/or take a handful of supplements every day and you don't like the fact that you will "need to do this forever"—and

you will—or if it just doesn't feel right, or you are concerned about the long-term health consequences of these programs, read on.

You have tried all of the diet, drug, vitamin, and exercise crutches and they either have not helped, have helped only a little, or you have found that while doing them, new symptoms have emerged that concern you, and you get that maybe you need to change your path.

You need to lose weight and are ready to take the time to do it right; you are ready to stop blaming yourself for your weight problems; and you are ready to focus on your health and hope that your weight will improve as a result, it will!

You know and believe that things can be better, easier, and different, read on. If you want to become incredibly educated and empowered about your health, read on. If like me, doctors have told you that there is no cure for your condition or disease, but you are not ready to accept this, read on.

Based on Years of Personal and Professional Experience

When I was ill and returned to school to study for my Masters of Science in nutrition, I completed courses in the sciences that gave me the needed foundation to understand how to heal the body. I also spent numerous hours reading about healing and worked for chiropractors, nutritionists, and a homeopath. Approximately two years into the master's program, when I realized that this degree would give me credibility, but not the knowledge, I needed to help others heal, I left the program and completed my bachelor's of science in nutrition with an alternative school and became certified as a nutritional consultant.

I started working in southern California sixteen years ago and then moved to Boulder, Colorado. I have been here for the last fifteen years where I have maintained a very successful private practice. I work with local clients as well as many clients from all over the country and a few from other parts of the world. I have accomplished this success for over fourteen years solely through client referrals. All together, I have over twenty years of personal and professional experience in health and healing, and I estimate I have spent over 30,000 hours figuring out how to heal the bowel and body.

House building 101

This program is based on sound principles of physiology and chemistry. In my private practice, I prefer to use analogies than technical lingo. Clients find this information much easier to understand this way, which facilitates success. I will do that in this book as well.

I will refer to your body as though it were a house in need of remodeling. All of you have a house that needs improvements and updating. Even if your house was originally built with low quality materials, these can be replaced. If you inherited some genetic weaknesses, they can be changed. Before you begin your remodeling job you will hire a contractor. He will lie out the plans for you, give you a cost estimate, and these variables will be weighed, along with how you connected with the contractor. Did you like him? As you read this book, I hope you find that I am the contractor for you.

When you remodel your house you will be moving trash, old kitchen cabinets, dust, etc. out of the rooms that need work into your trashcan outside. If your trashcan is too small or if it has holes in it, you will have a mess when you throw trash into it. Your front yard will look horrible and you won't like it. If you rip off your old kitchen cabinets and there is no room for them in the trashcan, they may sit around the floor of your kitchen and you won't like that either. I will help you remodel your house so that a mess isn't made, and I will help you fix your trashcan so that future trash is eliminated.

If you hire workmen to do the remodeling and they keep canceling on you, you won't be happy with how long the job is taking, and will likely hire someone else. I will help you heal your body as fast as possible.

After some time and money, you should be thrilled with your new house. It should be more beautiful than you imagined possible. It should also last a very long time. This program will help these come true.

Others qualified to help you?

I almost didn't write this book because many of you will need additional support than this book can offer, from someone qualified, like me. I can only help so many people. I don't know others who have the knowledge in healing the bowel that I do, but I just couldn't keep waiting to write this and share this information. Hopefully, the worst-case scenario is that many of you will get on the right road and stay on it long enough to trust the process and stick to it. To assist you, additional books will be available. They have already been written. When I set out to write this book and share my knowledge with you, it didn't occur to me that my small font, single-spaced, Word document would translate into a much larger book. Once this was done I found myself with a 900 page book (and to think I was actually limiting my writing!) To make this manageable I have broken this down into three books and will have the others available as soon as possible. They will greatly assist you with this process.

My vision includes training other professionals in this work. I believe this book needed to be written before this was to happen. If the demand exists, the supply will come. Right now there is an enormous demand for crutches, and therefore there are many professionals able and willing to recommend them to you. When you demand help in healing your bowel and body, professionals will respond and change their focus.

Watch out for defensive criticisms

You may hear critical or defensive comments about this book from medical or alternative health professionals. If so, this response is unfair (they have no experience or knowledge about the concepts I am sharing), childish, and incredibly selfish. You need to realize that these professionals do not know everything about health and healing. If you hear derogatory comments, you should consider finding someone to help you who is emotionally healthier, as his/her lack of emotional health will interfere with your ability to achieve your health and weight potential.

I have read thousands of health books, articles, industry publications, and magazines, and I have attended numerous lectures. I have always looked at this information from the perspective of how it supports healing the bowel. Much of what I have written is based on science, studies, and physiological knowledge, but I can in no way go back to the twenty years that I began this journey and document where it all came from.

This book may be ridiculed because there are very few scientific studies that prove what I am sharing with you. To this I *emphatically* state--**prove that I am wrong.**

I am still learning

This is a very different book than the one I would have written five, ten, or fifteen years ago. Recently I read a bestselling book about a man who had only a short time ago eliminated his intestinal symptoms and I thought, oh no, he wrote it too soon. He's going to realize that some day. If I had written this ten years ago, I would be changing my tune today, for although the approach has been the same, the skills and knowledge for best accomplishing this have changed a great deal in the last ten years. I've always wanted to write a book on my experiences and knowledge about healing, but deep down, I always knew that I wasn't ready. I now understand that I wasn't. I also now understand that most of *you* weren't ready for this yet, either. *You are now.*

I do not promise to have all of the answers and I suspect that, as has occurred over the years, I will find new, better, and faster ways to help people heal their bowels and bodies in the future. But I can promise that the general ideas, philosophy, and approach will remain unchanged. I will never and have never recommended a high protein diet as the solution, or large amounts of supplements that treat symptoms and do not heal, and I have and always will focus on healing the body by healing the bowel. I am open to learning as much as I can, and I am devoted to continuing my studies in this area and doing my best to share this word with others.

What do I gain from writing this?

Ultimately, I am writing this book because I feel like it is my responsibility to honor the unique knowledge and experience I have. *If someone criticizes this book or me, it is he or she who will be hurt, not me.*

It is emotionally disturbing to me when I read or hear about people who have suffered needlessly, as I did. It further inspires me to write and share these secrets and information. If people do not want to listen to it, so be it. At least I will have done all that I can to help. What I have to gain from writing this is the lifting of what has until now felt like a heavy burden of responsibility. I cannot move on in my life until this is complete.

Do you want to get results faster?

Contrary to all of the approaches to health and weight loss that use crutches and fail, there is no one magic food or supplement that will help you heal your bowel and body quickly. Others will try to convince you that there are, but this is factually untrue. Understanding the concepts of healing is your ticket to a smooth and quick ride down the healing road. Most, or all, of these concepts will be new to you. They require you to see things from a very different perspective, and it can take time and work to change this. To fully understand the concepts and perspective given in this book, re-read it over and over again until you do. This is the way to get results faster. It also improves your chance of success.

Schedule appointments/visit my blog

If after reading this, you would like to schedule an appointment with me so that I can personally help you, please contact me at donna@ThisWorksCrutchesDont.com, or 303-440-3559. If you would like to view my responses to your most common questions, my weekly reactions and thoughts about health and healing, and current status on upcoming books/seminars/etc., please visit my blog at www.ThisWorksCrutchesDont. blogspot.com. Also, look here if you leave me a phone message or email and I do not respond within 72 hours. This will only happen if I am out of the country, or I am unable to handle the demand for this information, in which case I will keep you updated on my blog.

Chapter One

How This Program Works

A Quick Summary of the Main Concepts

This Works is a unique book based on experiential knowledge stemming from the accumulation of sixteen years of work helping clients heal their bowels and bodies. It describes a program that I developed and refined over these years, a program that cured me of my "incurable" autoimmune disease, alcoholism, and food allergies—when all else had failed. The majority of information in this book is original and I am not aware of its existence anywhere else.

***This Works* teaches you how to heal your bowel. Currently, neither conventional nor alternative medicine offers programs that do this. No client has ever walked into my office with health and/or weight complaints who had a healthy bowel.**

When my clients heal their bowel, all symptoms, illness, disease, addictions, and weight problems go away—even the most difficult, critical, and stubborn ones. All symptoms, including those that one might think are inevitable due to mental stress, food allergies, old age, genetics, or any other cause, are eliminated. My clients who heal their bowels do not get cancer, heart disease, osteoporosis, diabetes, or any other illness. I am not aware of any other program that can deliver these results.

Relying on crutches—vitamins, drugs, exercise, food allergy diets, low carbohydrate diets, low calorie diets, alkaline diets, fasting, detoxification programs, laxatives, enemas, chiropractic, acupuncture, alcohol, recreational drugs, nicotine and all other addictive substances, etc.—to look and feel great will always *fail you. Stop blaming yourself.*

Crutches fail you for many reasons, but some of the most notable include the fact that you may miss an important one. This can be dangerous, or deadly. Putting a tarp over your roof that has holes in it but missing the section over your bathroom can cause your bathroom to flood when it rains. Crutches fail you because it is difficult and annoying to have to depend on these forever.

When you get tired of using them, you are back to your original problems and the search for a different, easier, better crutch ensues. It is the next great diet, or magic vitamin from an exotic, remote island in the sea! And as time goes by, stronger and stricter crutches are often needed to get the same symptom and weight reduction results, at levels that become near impossible to stick with. For example, to lose weight or feel better you may have to completely eliminate all carbohydrates, exercise obsessively, or ingest a huge quantity of vitamins everyday. With crutches, you are given a false sense of security. They are dangerous because they can make you believe that you are healthier, and safer, than you really are. **Feeling good and/or looking good because you use these crutches does not mean that you are healthy and have lowered your risk of illness and early death.** It also does *not* mean that you have healed your body, as many proponents of these claim.

This book will help put you on the right track and give you the tools needed to eventually eliminate the need for all of these crutches. . **When you heal your bowel, you will look and feel great *without* these crutches.**

"It makes sense," is the most common reaction to this information that I hear.

A Healthy Bowel Eliminates Acids From Your Body as a Strong Trashcan Eliminates Trash From Your House

Your body is constantly working to maintain an internal balance, or homeostasis. It is particularly critical to keep your bloodstream in balance. Of all of the variables in your blood, like calcium, magnesium, and iron levels, the pH is the most critical. If it goes too low, death occurs. Diet, stress, environmental toxins, chemicals, drugs, and medications contribute towards an overly acidic blood pH. Acids in your blood also originate internally from old cells, as every day some of them are dying and being replaced with new, healthier ones.

To maintain your health and weight, these acids need to enter into your blood, move on to your lymphatic system, and then into your bowel to be eliminated. Just as we generate trash in our day-to-day living that has to be thrown out, so our bodies have this acidic trash that it needs to eliminate daily, too. (*Throughout this book I may refer to the bowel with the following relatively synonymous terms: gut, large intestine, colon, and intestine. While these are not technically the same—for example, the large intestine encompasses your cecum, colon, and rectum—for the purpose of simplicity I have taken the liberty of using these definitions loosely. Additionally, I may refer to acids with the following relatively synonymous terms: toxins, trash, and waste.)*

For the majority of you, these acids are not completely eliminated once they reach your bowel because your bowel is not healthy enough to do so. Constipation is discussed most often in this country and generally only those people who are constipated realize their bowel is unhealthy and that their poor elimination is negatively affecting them. **Yet, eight-five percent of my clients have daily, but poorly formed, stools. Like most of you, they harmfully and mistakenly believe that this is healthy. In this case, as in cases of constipation, few of the acids that reach your bowel are eliminated.**

If this trash or acidity does not get eliminated, it gets stored in your body. Storage results in weight gain, nutritional depletion, organ decay, and disease. How would you like to live in a house where the trash never gets taken out? For most of you, this is occurring in your body. *Un-eliminated acids* are re-absorbed into your lymphatic system and eventually into your blood stream, where they trigger reactions from your other organs to deactivate them to protect you from them. If this did not happen you would die.

The reactions of your organs to these un-eliminated acids create health and weight problems. Here are a few examples. Your body retains excess water and creates excess fat cells to dilute and buffer these acids. This protects you and your blood from becoming too acidic, but it results in weight gain and dehydration. Your body also buffers these un-eliminated acids with oxygen, resulting in lower levels. Insufficient oxygenation is implicated in fatigue, slow healing, anemia, cancer, poor circulation, asthma, and heart attacks and stroke, for example. Excess acidity also stimulates the production of excess insulin and cholesterol. Eventually, these un-eliminated acids become stored in your organs, waiting for a chance to escape. If enough of these are trapped in your cells, they eventually cause degenerative disease and death. A more complete explanation of this process and the consequences of these un-eliminated acids are presented in Chapter 4.

Starving, eating fewer carbohydrates, exercise, yoga, chiropractic adjustments, massage, medications, vitamins and other supplements, and all of the other crutches you use to look and feel better do little if nothing to heal your bowel and improve your body's ability to eliminate these acids more efficiently. This program heals your bowel so that these acids can be safely, quickly, easily, and permanently eliminated.

This program is desperately needed, because many of you are in danger. Un-eliminated acids in your blood trigger symptoms and weight problems: acids in your organs cause disease and death, but fewer symptoms and weight problems. When you eat a higher protein diet, more acids remain in your cells and fewer enter into your blood, making you look and feel better. Your blood cholesterol levels may go down, as the cholesterol clogging your arteries, which puts you at risk of a heart attack, goes up!

Many people on these diets are dangerously led to believe that they are healthier than they really are. When they get cancer five years later, they do not blame the high protein diet because they wrongly think they were healthy because they felt and looked good, and their blood tests were "normal." You hear this story all the time, of the thin and/or "healthy" person who "suddenly" has a heart attack or is diagnosed with cancer. New studies are confirming this phenomenon, which I have seen and understood for many years.

Recently a client revealed that she knows fifteen people in their forties and fifties who are battling cancer. When I asked her what they look like, a shocked expression came across her face as she realized that 100% of them are thin and look fit. *Being thin and fit does not necessarily mean you are healthy.* **This program creates a body that is thin, fit, *and* healthy. In this program, the acids do not have to be "shoved" from your blood into your cells for you to look and feel good; instead, they exit your bloodstream and are eliminated by your bowel.**

Likewise, a high fiber diet moves acids from your blood into your bowel. This too is healthy and desirable, but it produces gas, loose stools, and discomfort if your bowel is unhealthy. These reactions cause many of you to abandon these healthy diets. Also, if these acids cannot be eliminated once they reach your bowel, they become re-absorbed and therefore the fiber does not "work." The promise of weight and cholesterol reduction that comes with eating a high fiber diet, for example, does not manifest.

When your bowel is healthy, a high carbohydrate, high fiber diet produces zero discomfort or weight gain. Ultimately, as all of the valid, long-term research has shown, this also dramatically extends your life.

"Eliminox" versus detox

Numerous natural "cures" and supplements promise to detoxify your body. This program is significantly more effective and very different from most detoxification programs, and for this reason I have coined the term "*eliminox*" to describe this program's process. *This program is designed to do what detoxification and cleansing programs don't, which is eliminate old toxicity/ acidity and heal your bowel so that it can help with this job, as well as ensure that this job continues to be done effortlessly and effectively in the future as well.*

Most detoxification programs are simply comprised of a bunch of supplements, like Milk Thistle, that help your unhealthy liver bind acids so that you feel better, but they do nothing to help *eliminate* the acids that *cause* your unhealthy liver. Taking supplements that bind to acids so that they do not cause discomfort is not the same as eliminating these acids permanently from your body in the first place.

If you take a supplement or do a program that promises to detoxify and heal you, but your bowel movements do not improve in frequency and form while doing this, you have not increased the elimination of acids from your body.

Healing should be safe and comfortable

Cleansing programs can cause acidic toxins to be released from your organs into your bloodstream and bowel. It is the inability of your bowel to eliminate these that causes the discomforts associated with some of these programs. Sometimes an excessive amount of acids are released from your cells into your blood, triggering loose stools and subsequently, electrolyte imbalances and dehydration. This is uncomfortable and potentially dangerous.

Additionally, when these acids are not eliminated, they are reabsorbed and settle back in your organs, where they came from. So not only do you feel bad, but no positive health improvement comes from it! Ouch. That is very hard to accept, I know. Too many people wrongly assume that this discomfort is productive and something one has to go through, but this is definitely not true. *With my program, you should never feel worse because of it.* If you had to feel bad to become healthier you might need to somehow learn to deal with it, but *healing should not be uncomfortable. If it is, it is wrong.*

Don't we detoxify naturally?

A recent statement that criticized detoxification and cleansing programs said, "We have systems to eliminate toxins naturally, so we don't need help." I agree. You *should* be able to eliminate naturally, but when your bowel is unhealthy, this doesn't happen and you can no longer rely on your natural systems. With a healthy bowel, as created in this program, you *won't* need to do something all the time to keep your body free of toxins. When you are finished healing your bowel, then, and only then, will you have the natural ability to detoxify your body without further help.

Healing Your Bowel

Your bowel is home to 100 trillion bacteria. A healthy bowel contains a large percentage of "good" bacteria, and an unhealthy bowel contains a large percentage of "bad" bacteria. When there are too few good bacteria, your bowel cannot eliminate acids sufficiently; there are "holes in your trashcan."

Rebuilding the internal bacterial environment of your bowel heals it; it fixes these "holes."

Healing your bowel is entirely different from cleansing it, using laxatives, taking fiber like psyllium, or doing enemas and colonics. These do not heal your bowel. Neither does a healthy diet, exercise, yoga, or 99% of the supplements and crutches that people use.

In addition to eliminating the acids that cause symptoms, illness, disease, addictions, and weight problems, your good bowel bacteria are vitally important for other health and weight functions too. These bacteria help prevent bacterial infections like strep, sinus infections, pneumonia, and E-coli. They help regulate hormones like estrogen and testosterone. When your bowel is unhealthy, excess estrogen is reabsorbed. Most, if not all, cases of breast cancer are caused by excess estrogen. I have worked with a number of women who had spent a lot of time and money taking supplement crutches from their naturopath, etc. only to be diagnosed with breast cancer later on. This never happens to my clients when they have healed their bowel. *They never get breast cancer.*

Your bowel bacteria help you digest gluten and lactose so you do not have allergies to wheat and dairy, they reduce sugar cravings, and they produce chemicals, similar to anti-depressants, which improve your mood. Most addictions are eliminated when these chemicals are balanced with this program. Your bowel bacteria also help with the production of numerous nutrients and enzymes you need to feel and look great and live a long life. A complete description of the functions of your healthy bowel bacteria, and the necessity to heal it, is given in Chapter 4.

An individualized, safe, and aggressive approach

It is impossible to quickly reverse the negative effects of decades of genetic, dietary, environmental, and mental stressors that cause an unhealthy bowel simply by improving your diet. To heal your bowel, you need to take very aggressive, safe, *temporary*, individualized amounts of products to rebuild the beneficial bacterial environment in it. In my practice, **this is done with my private** label product called *Bowel Strength,* or with extremely high, and therefore effective, amounts of probiotics, like acidophilus.

I have many years of experience with this and have yet to meet someone else who does, too. While some practitioners recommend probiotics, and some people have added them in on their own, *I have never seen anyone who was using ones that were individualized or nearly aggressive enough to work.* **Quick healing is a necessity for one to achieve success.**

For example, I have young clients under the age of ten who have seen dramatic improvements and relief from difficult conditions like autism, A.D.D., hepatitis, Tourett's, and Inflammatory Bowel Disease, by taking 400 billion organisms or more of probiotics every day for two to three years. In comparison, other programs may recommend 3 billion organisms a day (and this is almost always coupled with a high protein diet). At that rate, it could take two hundred years or longer to heal their bowel and body. In other words, it is completely ineffective. (Not to mention the fact that the bowel healing properties of this mere 3 billion organisms a day is offset by this bowel-weakening, high protein diet anyway!)

My knowledge and experience is that *it is the proper application of these supplements, and not the supplements themselves, that produce remarkable results.* You may buy the exact paint that Picasso used, but that does not mean that you can produce a painting that looks like Picasso's! You may buy the best quality bowel-healing supplements that the world has to offer, *but that won't mean anything unless you use them correctly.* This book will teach you how to use these so that you achieve maximum results.

Supplements that heal your bowel and body are very different from crutches, and must be used very differently. These concepts are also explained in *This Works.*

Bowel misunderstandings lead to failure

Most of you have never had a discussion with your doctor, or even alternative health practitioner, about the frequency and form of your stools. Wrongly, many of you think you are eliminating fine. Numerous misconceptions about the bowel lead to this way of thinking and prevent you from achieving your health and weight goals. These are addressed and explained in *This Works.*

The greatest misunderstanding about the bowel has to do with the frequency of elimination. Most of you have wrongly been told that the more often you go, the more waste you are eliminating. The physiology of your bowel and how stools are formed is described in this book so that you understand why this isn't true. Then, and only then, can you be successful with the recommendations I make.

Your bowel can be unhealthy even if your bowel movements are good

Occasionally I see a client who, during the course of our initial consultation together, incorrectly comments that their bowel movements are regular and well-formed and therefore their weight, symptoms, addictions, and/or disease cannot be due to an unhealthy bowel.

The reason for the above misunderstanding is because the form and frequency of your elimination by itself does not guarantee that your bowel is healthy. If you have holes in your trashcan but you never throw trash into it, you may think that your trashcan is fine, too. If your bowel is unhealthy but you eat a lower carbohydrate or lower fiber diet, very little acidity, or trash, will make its way into your bowel and you can wrongly think that your bowel is much healthier than it really is, too. Because so many people are now eating low carbohydrate, low-fiber diets, many people dangerously believe that their bowels are healthier than they really are.

I have yet to work with someone who has a healthy bowel when they come into my office, and I have yet to work with someone who doesn't feel and look better once their elimination improves. I am positive that all of you who work hard to maintain your weigh, have symptoms, addictions, or an illness have an unhealthy bowel. Never once over the years have you been told how to fix your bowel. This book provides this answer.

Crutches Are Used Temporarily

If you break your leg a pair of crutches will prove very helpful until your leg heals. Without them, you may be stuck on the couch for a while. With them, you can get up and move around more easily. There are still, however, great limitations to what you can do when your leg is broken and you use these crutches. You can't go running or skiing. You may not be able to drive very well, and you certainly can't take a shower with the same ease as before. Using the crutches is better than not, but a healthy working leg is best.

The crutches that you use when you break your leg are not helping your leg heal; they are simply helping make your life easier until it does. The same mentality holds true for the crutches available for feeling and looking better.

They have a purpose, which is to help you look and feel better until your body is healed and able to maintain these results on its own. At the same time, when your bowel and body are healed, you will look and feel better than you did when you were using them.

Healing your bowel takes time. Rebuilding 100 trillion bacteria to a healthy level is a monumental job, even with the very aggressive healing agents used. *This Works* provides information on how to use crutches safely, effectively, and temporarily while healing your bowel and body. This may include the *short-term* continuation of a higher protein diet and easy dietary changes, vitamins, physical modalities like acupuncture and chiropractic, and even pharmaceutical drugs. These crutches can help you immediately look and feel better, giving you the faith and patience needed to succeed with healing your bowel and body. If symptoms are not quickly improved, you will stray off the healing road. You will look for a quick fix, and fail.

I have a wealth of experience and knowledge in using crutches to safely help you look and feel better while you are healing your bowel. Many clients arrive at my door using crutches that are not working. I will help you find ones that do. My clients are more open to this information when they understand that these recommendations are intended and only helpful in the *short-term*. Some very valuable crutches are highly unused due to a lack of comfort, trust, and knowledge about them. Like drugs, many people are rightfully suspicious of taking supplements in the long- term. With the understanding of how their body works and the effects of an overly acidic blood pH, my clients are much more likely to use crutches and succeed doing so.

The Diet Part Is Easy

I think the number one reason people fail to improve their health is because of the fear of having to change their diet. Deep down they know, as did I when I was ill, that they would fail in this attempt. Yet, **what you eat is much more a product of the imbalances in your body than your knowledge, intentions, discipline, or willpower.**

My diet used to be atrocious—mostly refined carbohydrates, alcohol, sugar, and animal protein. When I became ill I knew my diet needed to change and I desperately wanted to eat better, but I hated fruits and vegetables and I ate the foods I craved. I knew they weren't good for me. I wanted to eat healthier, of course (everyone wants to have a healthy body and treat it right); I just couldn't do it. Many of you are in a similar boat. You don't need me to tell you that your sugar, coffee, alcohol, meat, etc. are not good for your health.

You need your body to tell you that for you. My body does that now, and yours will too as you follow this program.

This program will change your internal chemical balance. For example, excess un-eliminated acids reduce the production of enjoyable chemicals to your brain. They also lower your blood sugar, both of which can make you tired and depressed. Many foods act like drugs and alter your brain chemistry and blood sugar. When your bowel is healthy and eliminating acids efficiently, your desire for these "drug-like" foods—like sugar, animal protein, alcohol, coffee, and nicotine— is minimized, and often completely eliminated. I realize this is hard to believe. All of my clients look at me with skepticism when I announce this. But it does occur. Clients who swear that they will never give up hamburgers do. When they swear they will die without their coffee, they give it up, and feel better than they did when they needed it. Oh yea, I know, you say that you just love the taste of coffee, or the ritual that goes with it, but there is an underlying chemical reaction that occurs when you drink it that makes you feel good. *Ultimately, we are all craving that "feel good feeling."* When you are healthier and feel good because of it, you will no longer need coffee to achieve this, and you will find it unappealing to you. I understand if you don't believe this. I wouldn't have either many years ago. I now *crave* healthy foods that twenty years ago, I would have bet any person a million dollars I would never eat. And my favorites, diet soda and alcohol, disgust me now. Follow this program and be amazed when it occurs to you too. Everyone else always is.

This effect will assist you in making healthier dietary changes along the way. This reaction is one reason why this program is desperately needed. Without it, many of you will struggle and fail at ever maintaining a healthy diet long-term. All of you want to eat well, and this program will make that happen easily. **In the end, you will crave a healthy diet and your fear and confusion around food will be eliminated.**

This is not a book on vegetarianism. The *end* result of healing your bowel and body is that you will crave very little animal protein (beef, chicken, fish, turkey, etc.), and feel and look great eating this way, regardless of your blood type, close resemblance to cavemen, or any other reason you have been sold on high protein diets! But this is the *end* result. If you eat a high carbohydrate diet now, before your body is healthier, you will feel and look worse and fail to heal your body. I get this. In most cases I make sure my clients do not immediately give up their meat and eat more carbohydrates. *Eventually* they get to a place where they desire less animal protein; a place that all of the studies show will help you live much longer; a place that has more positive impact on the health of our planet than anything else you can do.

Finally, your current physiological weaknesses will be respected, and the diet recommendations will reflect this. For example, if you are allergic to dairy, do not add this back into your diet until your body can tolerate it. **When your bowel is unhealthy, it is impossible to make drastic healthy dietary changes, including the adoption of a healthy high carbohydrate diet if you are currently avoiding or limiting them, and feel good doing so. It is also unnecessary. Dietary changes in this program are gradual and extremely easy to follow.** This book outlines a transition diet plan to follow while healing your bowel and body. **Ultimately, your healthy body will cause you to feel great and lose weight, not a strict diet.**

Can This Program Help Me with My Condition?

Are there limits of this work? I don't know. But when someone comes in with a new condition I have never seen, this is much less complicated than you might think. **I believe that if you focus on healing your bowel and body, the possibilities are, astronomical, and endless.**

Some of the most common conditions that I have worked with and that have been eliminated with this program are: aches and pains, acne, A.D.D., adrenal fatigue, alcohol and drug addictions, allergies, anemia, arthritis, asthma, autism, autoimmune diseases like chronic fatigue, lupus, fibromyalgia and multiple sclerosis, bacterial infections, bloating, bronchitis, cancer, Candida, Celiac, colitis, constipation, Chron's, cystitis, diabetes, diarrhea, difficulty gaining weight, eating disorders, eczema, fatigue, fibroids, food allergies, fungal/parasite infections, gas, gluten intolerances, gout, headaches, heart disease, hepatitis, high cholesterol, high or low blood pressure, hypoglycemia, infertility, insomnia, lactose intolerances, lowered sex drive, osteoporosis, overweight, psoriasis, thyroid problems, viral infections, and water retention/edema. I personally had many of these problems, which have been completely eliminated.

This list is not to be interpreted as all-inclusive and representative of the only ones this program can help. I have also worked with people with a number of other symptoms as well as very complicated diseases and conditions that were called "medically incurable."

In my early experiences with alternative health I was diagnosed with Candida and Epstein Barr Virus (now more commonly referred to as Chronic Fatigue.)

I read all the books I could find on these two problems and attended some support groups meetings for Chronic Fatigue as well. My focus was on "treating" these conditions. It took a lot of failures and education before I realized that if I were healthy, I wouldn't have these conditions, and my focus should therefore be on getting healthy! This may seem very obvious, but many of you have done the same thing—focusing on your symptoms or weight rather than on your health. Sure enough, with my new focus, I was led down a better path. I got off the path of programs that relied on crutches. I stopped looking for the quick fixes, because I realized that it takes time to become healthy.

The realization that I should focus on getting healthy, and trust that my symptoms and illness would go away, was a turning point in my healing process. It led me to the complete and permanent elimination of my current and past symptoms.

A greater understanding of the physiology behind many health conditions, addictions, illness, diseases, and weight problems is presented in *This Works, Crutches Don't 2*. For now, **regardless of your condition, trust that if you focus on healing your bowel and body, it will go away.**

It is Not Hard to Do

The majority of my clients describe this program as very easy to do. You do not need to take handfuls of supplements every day for many years, you do not need to engage in colonics or any other therapy that is commonly undesirable, and you do not need to force dietary or other changes that will make you look and feel worse, or that will be difficult if not impossible to follow with success.

This program's difficulty lies primarily in the fact that it requires you to have a new perspective about your health and body. It can be hard, and take some time, to reverse ideas and thoughts that have been long established. You must read this book—maybe many times—and try to grasp the concepts and instructions given within. The ideas are complicated; the actions you need to take to make them work are not. You must trust this program, but what is often even more difficult, is the need to trust your body. Most of you don't, for good reason. You have to be patient. You have to be strong, as others will surely try to manipulate you to veer off the healing road. Your life will change dramatically as you do this, and while this is 100% positive, even positive change can bring some stress.

Ultimately, it is significantly more difficult to live a life filled with fear and discomfort than it is to heal your bowel and body, which will eliminate your fears and discomforts.

I am a "Billionaire"—You Can Be One Too

Thousands of dollars are spent every year on health insurance, new clothes, psychotherapy, trips to the "crutch" practitioner, and other expenses to treat the depression and discomfort of being overweight or not feeling well. How much does a lack of energy at work effect your productivity and paycheck? My health insurance costs me $120 a month. I'm with a very reputable company, but my rates are low because I never need to use it! How much do you pay? The number one cause of bankruptcy in this country is due to illness, and it happens often. I have never had a client declare bankruptcy as a result of healing their bowel.

Can you put a price on fear, or disease, or dying too young? How about having children? As the commercials say, "it is priceless." You spend $10,000 a month to try to get pregnant and $25,000 a month for addiction treatments. You have spent billions on weight loss crutches. Just for a chance for an outcome, but no greater health. In fact, often it is worse due to the treatment. When you do get results they are temporary, but you usually think it was "worth the money" because of the immediate benefit received. This causes a lot of problems, and leads to short-term, quick fixes that do nothing to help make you healthier. Unfortunately, when the problem comes back—and it will— you usually don't think you wasted your money, but you should. You do not think it was wasted because you always, wrongly, blame yourself, and not the program for your failure. So you spend thousands of dollars for programs that do not deliver long-term results, or prevent more serious problems in the future.

It is *significantly* less expensive to heal your bowel and body than it is to constantly treat your symptoms with drug, diet, and supplement crutches.

Saving for retirement

When you heal your bowel and body you will have no immediate indication that this is occurring. If you have 20,000 holes in your roof and fix 100 of these, you will not notice a difference. It will take time, and you might be suspicious and doubtful when things are not obviously being fixed right away and you are spending money every month.

When you embark on this program, think of it as an investment in your future. If you want to retire in ten years you need to save money every month. This is money that otherwise could be spent on new shoes, cars, vacations, clothes, or dinners out. You save this money because you want to be able to enjoy retirement. The reward from doing this is not immediate; rather it reveals itself in the future. You don't want to have to worry about having enough money to buy groceries when you are 75, and you don't want to have to work, either. When you heal your bowel and body and spend money doing so, you too are saving up for your future, a future free of discomforts, weight struggles, bankruptcy from illness, and/or premature death.

I am a billionaire—in spirit, physical, and emotional health. I would not trade all that I have in terms of my health, and knowledge of it, for all the money in the world.

There Is an End

This is not a quick-fix program. You can quickly look and feel better if you use the crutches recommended in Chapter 10, but you cannot quickly heal your bowel and body.

The length of time it takes to heal your bowel and body depends on the initial health of your bowel, the amount of stored acidity and subsequent weakness in your organs, and how quickly you choose to heal. It depends on how often you stop or get distracted along the way. If you stop at the Grand Canyon and numerous other attractions along the highway, and make wrong turns, it will take longer to get to the end of your journey than if you don't. One main intention of this book is to help reduce these distractions and help you heal your bowel and body as fast as possible.

This program has an end; ones that depend on crutches are *never*-ending. There are two paths you can take: One, depend solely on crutches and get quicker results but a lifetime of struggle, and a shortened life at that, or two, spend more time healing your bowel and body and gain the freedom from *ever* having to struggle or worry about your weight or disease again, as well as enjoy a long, healthy, enjoyable life. For me it is a no-brainer. Option number two is far preferable. I am offering that to you here.

Many clients get to the end of this program, while others get partway and decide it is good enough. This is up to you to decide. When your bowel is healed and you stop the program, symptoms that have been eliminated will stay eliminated for many years, if not forever, depending on how much healing, or remodeling, has been done.

At the end of this program, the *Bowel Strength* or acidophilus must be stopped. These products should never be needed again. Continuing to take them would be harmful. *This Works* guides you through this process.

Maintaining results with this program is simple. One, at the end of this program you will have "100 trillion healthy bacteria in your bowel," or "$100 trillion dollars in your bank." This would take a long time to spend, or damage again! What's more, you will find that you no longer desire the taste of many of the foods that at one time were appealing, and yet harmful to your bowel and body. Your healthier diet will help keep your organs strong.

Once your bowel is healed and your lifetime of accumulated acids have been eliminated, it would take decades for it all to go back to where it was, and even this is highly unlikely to happen.

At the end of this program yours stools will be perfect no matter what you eat, your weight will be effortlessly maintained, and you will be symptom-free. You will be healthier than ever before. You will crave healthy foods and not need to take extra supplements. You will look and feel great eating a high carbohydrate, healthy diet. You will realize that many of the symptoms that you put up with are not natural and are not a part of a healthy body. You will understand how excess weight, ill health, addictions, and disease develop. You will understand how you have reversed the process of disease development. You will feel utterly empowered and fear of weight gain and disease will no longer control you.

Give It a Fair Chance to Work—it Will!

Healing your bowel and body is an extremely complex, individualized process. Sixteen years of working with clients and thousands of hours spent trying to figure this all out has led me to a place where the technical aspects of healing have been simplified and made very clear. The greatest difficulty I have with clients involves helping them see their health and weight problems from an entirely new perspective. **Reducing fear, skepticism, feelings of powerlessness, confusion, misunderstandings, and impatience are keys to success.** This book aims to accomplish this.

This book is intended to put you on the right road with a very good idea of the road ahead and how to travel down it quickly, comfortably and effectively.

It points you in the direction of long-term success. Mostly, I wanted to help all of you who are heading in the wrong direction at 50 mph, reverse this and start heading towards health and healing.

When advice is geared to treat a symptom with a crutch it will keep changing, as it has many times over the years. When advice is given that helps make your body healthier, it won't. My advice to clients about their health has improved over the sixteen years that I have been consulting with them, but the main concepts and dietary philosophy have never changed, and I am certain they will not change in the next sixteen years either. The information in this book will stand the test of time. Its advice will be relevant and helpful for lifetimes to come.

This is not another book that simply repeats what others have said without unique experiences. Simply quoting a bunch of studies does not make one an expert on healing either. It is not a book, like so many others, that regurgitates information that others have discovered or stated. I read articles all of the time that give recommendations based not on an individual's own research and experience, but on what others have written in books, and in books that were written 20-30 years ago. I too read some fantastic books that were published over 30 years ago. They did not have the knowledge about how to heal the bowel, but they gave me a good foundation from which I have greatly expanded upon. Given our busier, more stressful lives, and declining health, it is more important than ever to adapt, improve upon, and add to the information provided many years ago so that the program is effective, fast, and doable.

I have discussed bowel health with every client I have worked with. On every visit the bowel is further described, respected, and discussed. For sixteen years my entire focus has been on figuring out how to effectively, quickly, and as easily as possible heal the body by healing the bowel. Every book, article, and other information on health and nutrition that I have heard or read has been looked at from the perspective as to how it can contribute to this model of healing.

This is not a book that gives ten easy and miraculous steps for alleviating symptoms and losing weight. If you need a quick fix, regardless of what it will cost you in the long run in terms of your health, wallet, or longevity, this is not the book for you. If you have tried numerous other approaches to lose weight or feel better and they have failed, I encourage you to read on. **I will help you to see how it is the approach that failed you; you yourself are not a failure.**

This is not another diet or something to try. I expect you to be a bit skeptical. I see skeptical clients all the time. I understand. I've been there too. Yet, many of my most successful clients, and those who refer me the most new clients, are ones that were the most skeptical, fearful, and unhealthy at the beginning of this program.

Healing your bowel and body takes time and you have to commit to it for a while. If you were going to a psychotherapist for counseling, you would not expect your emotional issues to be resolved in a month. You know that these things cannot change overnight. You must understand and accept that your physical being cannot be changed overnight either.

I urge you to give this program one year before you draw any conclusions about its benefit and ability to help you—when all else has failed. **Healing your bowel and body will never fail you.**

Chapter Two

How Did Everyone Get So Lost?

Most of you are zooming down the wrong road, and it is not your fault.

Your health and weight problems are not an inevitable product of stress, genetics, age, a lack of willpower, bad luck, etc. These are under your control.

You have been led down the wrong road by studies, blood tests, dangerous assumptions, misinformation, a harmful definition of health, and a lack of knowledge about how your body works and heals. You have been manipulated through fear. This program will help you take back your power and eliminate your fears. It will get you on the right road.

Hard to Hear, or a Blessing?

When I was ill, I spent thousands of dollars and many years deeply committed to other programs that didn't work. I wanted to believe that they benefited me more than they actually did. Many of you are in the same boat. I understand. It is very difficult to accept that you have been on the wrong road.

I had a new client recently who had spent $400 a month for six years on treatments and supplements from a Naturopath, only to get breast cancer. She was on a high protein diet and her bowel was extremely weak and nothing was being taken to strengthen it, which is a lethal combination. It was very difficult for her to accept that all of this time and money did not prevent her cancer. I was just told by a new client, a young woman with breast cancer, that she spent $50,000-$100,000 on alternative health care, that didn't work, prior to seeing me. Another new client spent fifteen years and $20,000 on alternative health care that left her worse off than when she started searching for an answer. She is bitter, angry, and suspicious. I hear stories like these constantly.

Sometimes I have clients who are out to prove I'm wrong because these experiences have jaded them, and hearing the truth is too difficult. It is very sad and unfortunate if you see your past journey solely in a negative, angry, pessimistic way. This attitude will ruin any chance of success for you.

If you are having difficulty with the idea that you have been heading down the wrong road, you need to gain a new perspective on it. *The roads you took may not have been the right ones, or the ones that led you to the end, but they were valuable roads, nevertheless.* They were the "beginning to the end." They helped you find, understand, and commit to the right road—this program—when you saw it. Rarely does a client succeed with this program that hasn't had a number of failures prior to it. When I was in sales there was a saying that it takes ten "no's" before you get a "yes." In this way, the "no's" weren't seen as negative, but rather as an inevitable positive to finally getting to the profitable "yes." You can view this situation in the same light. **The "no," or previous health or weight program that was wrong, can be seen as something positive that helped you get on the right path—this path.**

You did your best

There are several key reasons why I was able to heal my body from a devastating illness. One of these was that I never blamed myself for all of the wrong paths I took, both before I became ill and while I was searching for a cure. I have done a lot wrong in my life and have made many mistakes. But I did my best, and I saw these mistakes as beneficial; as something I could learn and become a healthier and happier person from. You have done your best too.

Up until now, the answers to your health problems, addictions, and weight problems have not been available to you. Your being lost, and your failures, is not due to a lack of effort, intention, or desire. **If your bowel and body are unhealthy, it is not your fault.**

If you are angry, frustrated, or in denial, replace this with a feeling of gratitude. This is hard to do, but your life will be much more difficult if you don't. Be grateful that an answer exists to your health and weight problems, at all.

The Crutches Aren't Working

We are spending more than half of all the health-care dollars in the world and yet people from 23 countries are living longer than us. For the first time in recorded history, cancer is the number one killer among 1-15 and 25-40 year olds. Lung cancer is now the most common fatal malignancy in men and women, and the incidence of lung cancer is rising each year. We are living in a time when cancer and heart attacks at age forty are not thought of as unlikely, and high cholesterol levels have been found in children as young as eight years old.

Asthma among children is now considered normal. My children know of at least six others who have asthma; whereas when I was growing up, I never knew a single person who had it. In the 1960s, one in 2,500 children was diagnosed with autism; today that number is one in 500.

Ten years ago 1:10 couples had problems with infertility; today that number is closer to 1:4. Twenty years ago, a baby born more than two weeks early was an anomaly. In many parts of the country today babies who are born early outnumber those who aren't. About seven years ago I had a client in Virginia whose neighbor had a baby. Nine out of the ten babies born that day at her hospital needed to be put in the I.C.U. That is an overwhelming number that we need to pay attention to.

Obesity is at an all-time high. We have more knowledge and are told the "answers" for losing weight, but we have completely failed to succeed with this information, because it is wrong. Diabetes, which used to be most prevalent among older adults, now inflicts millions of middle-aged Americans. In the fourteen years that I have been doing this work professionally, I have seen a noticeable increase in unhealthy bowels among children under ten years of age. This indicates the existence already of a very weak intestinal system and the corresponding potential for a quick accumulation of health-destroying acids in their bodies. I have witnessed an increase in unhealthy bowels among my adult clients as well.

The full effects of treating our health and weight problems with crutches like drugs, surgery, and high-protein diets have yet to be felt. That's the saddest part of it all. It will be another ten years or so before the damage is most prevalent. I strongly believe that unless we change things now, in ten years obesity, cancer, heart disease, asthma, infertility, and every other disease will be much greater than they are now, and much more common at much younger ages. Bill Clinton predicts that the current generation will be the first that does not out-live its parents. I agree. This program can prevent this from happening.

It's *not* About Genetics, Stress, Old Age, or Bad Luck

When someone walks into a medical office with a health or weight complaint, the issue is usually blamed on genetics, stress, age, or even bad luck. Many health and weight conditions that could be altered and eliminated are not being addressed because of the belief that these variables control your health and weight.

Your genetic inheritance is very relevant, but you have control over your genetic future and you do not have to be a victim to a poor inheritance. If cancer or heart disease runs in your family, for example, you can alter this vulnerability. If you inherited an unhealthy bowel, it can be healed.

The emerging field of epigenetics is showing that environmental influences can modify how genes function without actually altering DNA. Researchers have found that nutrients "generate chemical signals that act as genetic stop signs." They believe that if you make nutrition a priority when pregnant, for example, you may lower your child's inherited cancer risks.

Jack Challam, author of *Feed Your Genes Right,* notes that DNA and genes are not static blueprints, but rather dynamic software programs, constantly responding to what's going on in and around our bodies. That means if we eat junk foods, our genetic programming changes for the worse, and if we eat healthier foods, our genes function better.

There are numerous complicated, scientific explanations for why we can alter our genetics, but I prefer the following analogy: If your house was built with cheap windows, they can be changed. If you inherited a genetic weakness, it can be changed too. In both cases, however, action needs to be taken. It will not change by itself. This program will teach you how to replace those old, cheap windows with new, strong ones.

Genetics and your bowel

In the Spring 2007 *New York Times Style Magazine* I read about a new revolution of spas and doctors who are using genetic testing to help individuals measure the effect that their lifestyle choices are having on the rate of damage to their DNA. From there, individualized and aggressive dosages of nutrients are prescribed to try to offset this damage. While this approach uses crutches of mass vitamin supplementation and will ultimately fail, as I have seen all approaches that depend on these do, I was interested to read a comment by Dr. Andrew Cohen of the WellBeing Institute in which he described genetic damage in the following way:

"It's like a bathtub. The tub is your accumulated amount of DNA damage. So what controls that? There's the faucet: the rate of damage going in. That's stuff like smoking, sunbathing, eating pesticides. On the other end, there's the drain. That's your body's ability to repair the damage."

In this program, your bowel is the drain. Ultimately, what he is saying is that if you can eliminate this acidity/toxicity, your DNA will not become damaged! Having made this statement, I unfortunately found no evidence that his program includes healing the bowel.

This program heals your bowel so that DNA-damaging acids can be aggressively, safely, completely, effortlessly, and permanently eliminated.

He also mentioned that a third variable affects the damage to your DNA and ultimate chance of getting cancer and other ailments: sensitivity. He describes that as the height of the tub, which affects how quickly it will overflow. I would describe it as the inherited strength or weakness in your bowel from birth. A strong bowel from birth will eliminate acids longer than a weak or sensitive one.

(When your bowel is strong and eliminating well, it also makes sufficient quantities of vitamin B-12, and vitamin B-12 is needed to make and repair your DNA. A healthy bowel eliminates heavy metals like mercury and aluminum, preserving your zinc levels and reducing the genetic damage caused in part by low zinc levels.)

At least two lives

It would be lovely if we were like a cat with the fabled "nine lives," but we do have at least two. The human body is capable of amazing repair and regeneration. Roughly 300 billion new cells are created every day. Give them a healthy environment and they will be created more healthfully. Cells thrive in a non-acidic chemical soup. Eliminating acids by a healthy bowel helps create an environment conducive to healthy cellular growth.

I was given a second life, and daily I am grateful for this. You can have this too.

Squirrels are stressed out

A couple of years ago I went to see my favorite comedian, Bill Maher. During his monologue he spoke about how we like to blame stress for all of our health problems, but that many animals in the wild are faced with the same, or even greater stress, on a day-to-day basis, yet they have not become inflicted with the health problems that we have. He asked us to think about the squirrel, eating his nut, and constantly looking over his shoulder for a predator that may come and kill him. *That* is extreme stress. It makes you think….

Just because stress or any other variable may trigger a symptom does not mean that that variable is the cause of the problem.

If your roof has holes in it, your house will get wet when it rains. So the question is: Is the rain the cause of the problem, or the holes in the roof? Without the holes, the rain would not cause your house to become wet. The holes are the true cause of the problem. Healing your bowel eliminates these holes.

You can get younger as you get older

For most people, symptoms, weight gain, and disease are more prevalent as they get older because as one gets older, their bowel and body become less healthy. If you do not remodel your house, it too will wear down and become out-dated with age. My house, with its granite countertops, wood floors, updated sinks, and stainless steel appliances, looks better than it did when it was originally built thirty years ago. And at the age of 45, I am significantly healthier than I was twenty years ago!

It's not about bad luck

I read an article not long ago in which a woman in her 40's got breast cancer and believed it was "bad luck," since she was an avid runner. Running does not prevent cancer; a healthy bowel and body does. Running may make you look and feel better, but this is not the same as making your bowel and body healthy.

An article appeared in *People* magazine, August 30, 2002, about a baby born three months early and weighing only one pound. The mother had spent four years trying to get pregnant. After a miscarriage, she got pregnant again and delivered her baby three months too early. The doctor commented, "Jennifer (the mom) had no bad habits; she was just unlucky."

In my experience, any woman who suffers from difficulty to conceive (especially after trying for four years!) and then has a miscarriage has an unhealthy bowel, and a severely premature baby is not unlucky; it is a reflection of that mother's unhealthy bowel. When you heal your bowel, you greatly reduce your risk of delivering prematurely. The vast majority of my pregnant clients deliver within the week they are due. A few days ago another client had her first baby, and she was born only two days early. And this client originally approached me due to difficulties getting pregnant in the first place.

"Bad luck" is just a "bad bowel," and this can be changed

...Or our depleted soil, laziness, or toxic environment either

Yes, the environment is more toxic, our soil is more depleted, and we don't get our bodies moving enough. But this does not even begin to explain all of our health and weight problems. I see babies as young as three months old with very unhealthy bowels and health problems all the time. They have not lived long enough for the environment, stress, poor soil, or lack of exercise to harm them.

Survival of the Non-Fittest

Darwin's theory of survival of the fittest describes how in nature, only the strong survive. This helps to ensure that future populations are also strong and able to survive. **I strongly believe that the main reason rates of asthma, premature cancer and heart attacks, obesity, ADD, and other illnesses are on the rise is because we have manipulated this natural principle; we no longer have survival of the fittest working to ensure a population of strong, healthy bodies. The non-fittest are surviving, albeit not very well.**

In nature, there are not fertility clinics if a fox cannot reproduce; she simply does not have babies. *The inability to reproduce is a function of one's bowel and body health.* Infertility treatments force a woman to have babies when she is not healthy enough to do so naturally. In nature, a fox born too early, or with any complications, also dies. The healthier the mom and baby are, the less likely that a premature birth will occur.

Medical interventions at birth and infertility treatments are creating a generation of children that is less healthy and weaker than past generations. And these weaker children pass along weaker bowels and genes to their children, and so on. *In my opinion, these are the primary causes of the serious increases in ill health and obesity in this country over the last couple of decades.*

Additionally, long ago, before antibiotics, people with an unhealthy bowel, and subsequent inability to fight bacterial infections, would have died and been less likely to reproduce and pass this weakness on to their children.

None of my clients who have healed their bowels have given birth to a premature baby. Statistics show that very premature babies have a 25% to 30% chance of developing severe handicaps such as cerebral palsy and blindness, but what about the chance of less severe handicaps? I'm sure this is much greater. How about asthma, ADD, etc.? What about later in life? Are there higher rates of heart disease and cancer? Some scientists say "yes."

I do not criticize anyone for taking antibiotics, or using fertility methods to have children. If you were infertile you were told it "wasn't anything you could change," and you believed this, understandably. I believed all of the "experts" years ago who said that all you had to worry about was how many calories you ate, and drank gallons of acidic diet sodas believing I was not hurting myself. I get it; I "did this" many ways, many times. And if your baby was born early or needed medical intervention and is alive today as a result, thank goodness for that.

I have two children and I understand the yearning to reproduce. I am simply stating that infertility treatments and medical intervention at birth have caused an increasingly weak offspring with increasingly weak bowels, and an increase in health and weight problems as a result. An understanding of this is needed so that we can understand what is causing our problems and how to fix them. I am not in any way implying that these practices stop; but I am offering a program that will eliminate the need for infertility treatments and help babies stay in the womb until they are full term; a program that will dramatically increase the health of our babies and reduce the need for intervention when they are born; a program that will provide our future generations of children with healthier bowels, less obesity, and less disease.

I have successfully helped many clients get pregnant who couldn't before. Many clients get pregnant immediately upon trying. My children, conceived when I was in my 30s, are both the result of a single try. Neither of them was born early, and they were home births without complications.

If you used fertility methods to conceive, your baby was born more than a week early, or your baby needed medical intervention to survive, it is not too late to help him or her. It is highly unlikely that his or her bowel is healthy, but this is not a condition that you must accept. Following this program can change it.

And our future?

What is going to happen when all of these young children born in the past decade grow into their twenties and thirties? Will we see an increase in cancer and heart disease among them? Probably. Will it take this before we decide that we drastically need to change our approach to health? I hope not!

This is not unlike our response to global warming. For decades scientists have been warning us about the consequences of our lifestyles. But, we thought, not true, you are over exaggerating, and it is too much of a hassle to change our ways. What is it going to take before we realize we are in the same dire circumstances regarding our health? We have already experienced an unprecedented and alarming increase in cancer and heart disease among people younger than sixty years old. Over twenty years ago, when I was twenty, I didn't know a single person under sixty who had cancer or who had experienced a heart attack. Today I can rattle off a long list of names of people in this category. *Will we wake up when we start to see many people we know in their thirties getting cancer and heart disease? What is it going to take???*

Not long ago I watched the movie "Children of God." In it, women can no longer reproduce. Is this just science fiction, or is it an eminent reality? Will mothers who had difficulty getting pregnant, who were wrongly told it was "due to age," not ill-health, pressure their children to have children when they are younger, until even they are too unhealthy to reproduce? It may sound far-fetched, but is it really? I see extremely unhealthy twenty-year-olds all the time.

What happens when all of the children today who are being fed a high-protein, food allergy diet grow older? *For the first time in the history of mankind we have a large number of children being fed this way.* We've never experienced the dire, long-term consequences of this. But we will, one day in the near future, because these children have unhealthy bowels, and these diets accelerate cellular degeneration and disease.

Evolution of Health and Healing— —How Did We Get Here?

I am grateful that I became ill twenty years ago, at a time when healing the body was more prevalent then merely treating symptoms with crutches. (Although at the time, I thought the timing was horrific, as I was young, making good money, had a cute boyfriend, and wanted to play and party!) I spent hours upon hours in health food stores searching through books, trying to find the answer for my health crisis. I bought many of them. When I recently went to my local health food store to see what is currently available,

I was saddened and surprised to find that the vast majority of the priceless books I found long ago were not there.

The books I read long ago spoke of the importance of bowel movements. They offered remedies to cleanse and detoxify the organs with everything from colonics to apple cider vinegar drinks to baking soda and macrobiotic diets. They spoke of saunas and sunshine and fasting. The focus was *not* on taking a bunch of vitamins or drugs or following low carbohydrate diets. At that time, things were even much different in the medical field. When I was diagnosed with an autoimmune disorder, I was not given a long list of drugs I could use to feel better, as most patients are today.

The books I read back then were invaluable. They set up the foundation from which I would later build from and figure out how to heal the bowel and body. On the down side, many of these methods were uncomfortable, and very unappealing. They were time consuming, restrictive, and required a great deal of commitment and change, and many of them were perceived as strange and abnormal. On top of which, none of these approaches heal your bowel. Many of them are healthy (and much healthier than the high protein approaches of today), but most of them still do not help eliminate acids from your body and *none* of them fix the bacterial environment within your bowel, as this program does.

So when a book was published in 1990 that abandoned these practices and instead offered an immediate improvement in one's symptoms simply by ingesting numerous vitamins and herbs, it is no surprise that it became a hit. But it also became part of a movement away from healing, a place that we are still at nineteen years later. Taking a bunch of supplements does not eliminate the acids that cause your problems, as the other books promoted. But these supplements gave us a quick, easy fix and we responded like crazy to this concept. The amount we have spent as a nation on vitamin supplements has skyrocketed over the last decade into the many billions. The supplement companies and health food stores have enjoyed this explosion as well. When this particular book first came out I lived in southern California, two blocks from one of their largest health food stores. The store prominently placed this book at the entrance of the store, and I watched as many customers walked around the store with the book opened to a symptom and a basket filled with supplements. I worked in a smaller health food store earlier on and knew that supplement sales were much more profitable for these businesses than food sales. These stores were ecstatic. Shortly thereafter, this large store, with about 25% of its space devoted to supplements, acquired a vacant space next to it, and proceeded to devote this entire space to supplement sales, effectively quadrupling their attention to the sale of them, and dramatically increasing their profits as well. *The supplement companies and health food storeowners, and others who sell supplements, have benefited from this approach, but you have not.*

We need to get back to healing the body and eliminating toxins, or acids, from it. My program has improved upon the older methods used to achieve this. Compared to twenty years ago, products are now available that will help you eliminate acids quickly without the need to fast or do numerous enemas; products that will allow you to heal your bowel bacterial environment at a *much* faster rate than before, so that this process is quick, and permanent. For example, when I was ill, acidophilus that came in a 100 million organisms per capsule strength was considered revolutionary. Today, I can purchase it with 100 billion organisms per capsule, an increase in strength of 1,000%.

Our use of drugs to treat symptoms has also grown exponentially. Our society has become more fearful, more impatient, and more addicted to the quick fix. It is self-perpetuating. The more we travel this road, the more overweight and ill we become, and these conditions lend themselves to greater fear and impatience and therefore greater chances that we will resort even more to the quick fixes of drugs and supplements, at larger amounts than before.

It is my intention to lead everyone back to healing their body. Everything in life comes full circle, and it is time that this does too. We are currently living with a major health and weight crisis, and we have the opportunity to stop it before it stops us. Like our current environmental crisis of global warming, it can be changed, and it has to be, *now.* One of the greatest harms to our ozone layer and environment is the production of meats, like chicken, beef, and turkey. In fact, the greatest threat to our ozone layer is the methane from animals raised for consumption, not the emissions from cars. A healthy body does not need to eat a lot of protein to look and feel great. So we desperately need to heal our bowels and bodies, for the sake of our planet, as well.

I believe that the following concepts embody the main reasons why you have gotten lost in your search for health: your focus on short-term versus long-term results; reliance on studies for health information; fear; you got stuck in a vicious cycle; the accepted definition of health; and the accepted definition of success.

Long-Term versus Short-Term/ The Quick Fix

You have allowed success to be defined in the short-term, and this has led you to choose paths that deliver short-term success but long-term failures. Numerous books and programs claim to heal you or fix your health or weight problems, but this is always measured in the short-term. A recent bestselling book claims to have healed someone after only forty days. But where is this person in 400 days, or 4,000 days? *Practitioners fail time and again to share long-term stories. I see people with short-term success and long-term failure all the time. In every case, their bowel is weak. It was never fixed.*

Books are written all of the time by people who have no long-term, personal experience in the field. Most are written by people who have tried a "treat the symptom approach with crutches" who are feeling or looking better, and have rushed off to write about it, without any long-term experience and success with it.

Abstinence from a drug, alcohol, or sugar for one month is not success. Losing weight after one month of working with a personal trainer is not success. The reduction or elimination of symptoms or weight for one or two years is not a big deal. How about five or ten years? When a program can deliver those results, then it is a program worth considering.

There are many diet and health programs that can help you look and feel better immediately, but many of these make your body less healthy in the process, so that in the long-term you are worse off for having done so. Unfortunately, you never request long-term results from these programs, and because of this, you keep choosing ones that are bound for failure. Do you think that your neighbor failed to keep her weight off, or died of breast cancer, in the long-term, but you won't, on the same program, because you are "better than her?" *When a program fails, it is because the program is wrong, not because the person is wrong, or weak, or "less of a fighter" than you.*

Just because you look or feel better does not mean you are healthier! And it takes a healthier body to maintain your weight, live a long time, and be symptom-free in the long-term.

You can justify anything

Books that deliver short-term results have a clever way of justifying their advice. For example, in the book mentioned above the author justifies his high-protein dietary advice by saying that we had no osteoporosis long ago when we ate a lot of meat. But the fact is no bone density tests were done then, so we really don't have data on this, and this statement should not be made. Also, long ago we had minimal or no medical intervention, so only the healthiest lived, and the healthier you are, the less likely you are to have osteoporosis.

Testimonials create problems too

When a health professional uses testimonials to sell their approach, they are taking advantage of your desire for a quick fix. All of the testimonials that I have ever read are based on very short-term results. It is hard to get a client to write one of these, even if they have had remarkable results. But to follow up with a client many years later to obtain one of these, is extremely difficult, expensive, and simply not done. This is unfortunate, because *a long-term testimonial is the only one that you should give credence to.* If someone took a bunch of supplements and felt better one month later, that result is irrelevant. How about ten years later? Did this person have a reoccurrence of their symptoms? Were they worse? Did they develop a new condition or disease? Are they even still alive? These are the results that should impress you and guide you, not short-term ones.

Additionally, how credible are these testimonials anyway? Does anyone every check their validity? Are they real, or made up? Just the other day I received an email from a company that sells book-promoting tools. One piece of advice they gave was for the author to write their *own* testimonials and then try to find someone to sign their name to them!

Until testimonials can be obtained that can be validated and reflect long-term results of ten years or more, ignore them.

I have not desired or drunk alcohol for over twenty years. My autoimmune disease has been gone for over a decade. I eat a high carbohydrate diet, do not avoid wheat or dairy, and I do not take vitamins to maintain this. I am writing this book after personally having had long-term success with this program. If you are going to follow someone's advice, this is the long-term success you need to look for.

Studies are Dangerous

Research studies can be very misleading, and many are insignificant. Many studies look at a population of less than 100 people over only a few months of time and then attempt to draw some important conclusion. You cannot do this with nutrition because it takes nutrition many years to affect, negatively or positively, the health of your body. Yet it is done all the time and the majority of the reports and advice that you hear on the news, or from your doctor, are from studies that are absolutely irrelevant. *As a wise health consumer, you want to find out more details on a study before you accept the advice given from it.* The first variables to analyze are sample size and length of study. A study should last at least ten years and include at least 1000 people to be of any value and significance. Most studies do not meet these requirements.

Some people fail to heal their body because they give way too much credibility to studies and "need these" to trust the information they are given. This leads to failure because *studies are geared towards treating symptoms with crutches,* and you will not attain a long life and weight stabilization with this approach.

Very little of my work has been studied. But bear in mind, **the lack of a study simply means it has not been done, *not* that there is no relevant correlation.**

Hypocritically, only one-third of interventions used by conventional medicine are supported by randomized controlled trials, yet when nutritional protocols are suggested that have not been proven, conventional doctors tell you "they aren't proven, so don't bother using them."

They can never really isolate just one variable

A recent study reported that eating mega fruits and vegetables doesn't reduce cancer. What about other variables that were not controlled, or mentioned? For example, were these people eating more protein than they needed? If so, the cancer reducing benefits of eating a lot of fruits and vegetables would be "cancelled out" by the protein consumed. Also, fruit and vegetables are not as concentrated as supplements, and it can take decades for a healthier diet that contains more fruits and vegetables to positively affect your health.

Even the placebo control group that is a standard among most studies is fraught with problems. The sugar pills that people are given are not a real control; sugar affects the physiology of your body.

They lack key variables

You cannot in good conscience ask people to do something potentially harmful. Dangerous studies are conducted on mice and non-humans, but they do not have the credibility of ones that are conducted on humans.

If someone wanted me to conduct a study about my program I could not possibly have a control group that did something, like eat a high protein diet, that I knew could harm them.

31

Untrustworthy results and the politics of it all

The results of studies are often biased, false, and manipulated, depending on who profits. A recent report from UCSF researchers, who analyzed 200 studies of prescribed cholesterol-lowering drugs, or statins, found that the *results were twenty times more likely to favor the drug made by the company sponsoring the trial.*

A recent study found that eating fried food might increase your risk of obesity. No kidding! Who is wasting our tax money on these studies, and who is making money off of them? Other recent studies found that drinking soda may be bad for you! Eating a lot of ice cream may make you overweight! I can think of dozens of studies that would be worth our hard-earned money, but these aren't the ones getting done. Why not?

The same studies over and over again

There are thousands of studies on the benefits of antioxidants, found in tea, grapes, fruit, vegetables, vitamins A, C, E, and selenium, for example. (By the way, these help buffer the acids that your bowel is too unhealthy to eliminate.) But back to the main issue: Why do we need fifty short-term studies measuring the same variables?

The medical profession acts as though they are protecting you with all of these studies. "Well, gee, we know these antioxidants help your heart, but we haven't done studies yet to test if they are good for your diabetes. So don't take them for this until we, the great protectors, do a study to see if it will help it. We don't want you to waste your money for nothing." It could take decades before every condition is tested. If antioxidants are good for your heart, don't you think they could possibly help your diabetes, too? At the very least, you have to conclude there wouldn't be much harm in trying them.

Studies look at symptoms more than mortality

Most of the nutritional health studies that I read are geared towards treating symptoms with crutches. Most look at short-term and not long-term results, which are the ones that matter. Very few measure mortality. *A study may find that eating a high protein diet reduces cholesterol or blood sugar levels, but no one asks the more important question, "Did these people live longer?" It doesn't help you much to have low cholesterol or blood sugar if you are dead at age 55!*

I prefer analogies and physiological and biochemical education as a way to help you understand how healing your bowel will eliminate your health and weight problems. Many other health practitioners base much of their advice and education on nutritional studies. I will quote and comment on a few of these in this book, but for the most part, I find studies to be suspicious, at times very biased and misleading, lacking in their ability to help you understand your body as the whole, interrelated organism that it is, and completely useless in helping your understand how to heal your bowel and body and prevent health and weight problems.

Manipulation Through Fear

In the award winning documentary "Bowling for Colombine," by Michael Moore, the consequences of manipulation through fear are exposed. In response to the tragic shootings at Colombine High School, Moore set out to uncover the reason why we have so much more gun violence in America compared to other countries. His research uncovered the fact that in other countries—where gun possession is as high or higher than ours, where there is higher unemployment, equal amounts of divorce and lack of family support, equal teenage fascination with violent movies and video games, a past history of war and violence, and/or equal percentages of ethnic groups—far fewer people are getting killed by guns. In other words, he addressed, and shot down, all of the popular explanations given for why we had over 11,000 gun deaths in 2002, compared to only 60 or so in Canada or England, for example. *He points the finger at fear, a fear created by the industry that benefits from it and is then rapidly spread by the media.*

Moore concluded that we are kept in a state of fear and programmed to respond to it violently. The gun industry benefits from this enormously. This also benefits the politicians and their special interest groups who profit from this "we need to kill to protect ourselves" mentality.

This directly parallels the health industry in this country, as well. Most people who come into my office are suspicious of their body's ability to heal itself and be free of disease. I have helped numerous people, including myself, heal themselves from many symptoms and illnesses that we are told are incurable. Yet, it seems as though 99% of Americans believe this is not possible. It makes you wonder: *"Who profits from this?" It is definitely not you. It is not based on truth. The fact is you can heal your body.*

In 2004, major pharmaceutical companies spent almost $100 billion on marketing, yet only $50 billion on research and development. There are at least four pharmaceutical lobbyists for every member of Congress.

When was the last time you heard anything on prime-time news about someone healing themselves of an illness with alternative means? We have many television shows that glorify the medical profession: Grey's Anatomy, House, etc. Where are all of the shows about alternative healers? The media is extremely powerful and can manipulate millions of people in their thinking. Most of you likely don't know that you can heal your body because this is not depicted on television, and the books on healing have also virtually disappeared.

Of all the amazing physical and emotional benefits I received when I healed my body, by far the most rewarding was the elimination of fear. I used to be deadly scared of getting cancer, partly because two of my grandparents died at an early age from it. I had no idea that it was preventable. Had I not gone through this process, I would have also been afraid of the West Nile Virus (which was all over the news a few years back), AIDS, and that my children would die from polio if I didn't vaccinate them (which I didn't). Every latest health scare reported by the media would have frightened me. I also used to be constantly fearful of gaining weight. My fears are completely gone now, and my number one goal is to help empower you to feel the same way.

As sad as it is that forty or so people died from the West Nile Virus, it is also sad that millions of people responded by applying mounds of toxic insect repellent. This toxin is absorbed from your skin into your blood, where it weakens your immune system, the system that, ironically, is designed to help protect you from viruses like West Nile. *Ironically, many short-term efforts to eliminate the fear of disease create more stress in your body and make you more susceptible to the dangers of it.*

Recognize that your fear is unjustified. It has been put there to the advantage of others. You have a choice in your health care and you can decide to eliminate your fear of illness like cancer and premature death.

The Vicious Cycle

The greater your fear, the greater the pressure there is to get immediate results. Programs that provide immediate results come with a high rate of long-term failure, and this in turns leads to greater fear and a greater "need" to fix these problems quickly. A vicious cycle ensues.

Often I see new clients who have spent thousands of dollars on crutches that have failed, as they always do, and because of this, they are afraid to invest more time and money in this program. You will not succeed if you have this mindset and fear. This is not a quick fix program. It works. But it requires time and a commitment. It requires money, although much less than you will spend if you don't follow this.

More protein, less healthy bowel, and a greater "need" later on

A recent study conducted at Aberdeen's Rowett Research Institute in Scotland showed that a low carbohydrate diet can result in a fourfold reduction in the amount of certain types of beneficial bacteria in your bowel. These bacteria produce butyrate, which helps keep your bowel healthy and prevents colorectal cancer. *Researchers think that the healthy bowel bacteria need carbohydrates to produce this substance.*

In other words, if you are desperate to lose weight, you can easily fall for an unhealthy high protein diet and get some short-term results. This diet, however, makes your bowel less healthy over time, the organ that needs to be healthy for you to lose weight and keep it off permanently and effortlessly in the first place! By following this diet, you put yourself in a position where you will likely have greater future struggles with your weight. And when this happens, you may also be even more prone to look for a quick fix to this problem out of desperation. As your health goes down, impatience and depression go up, and this leads to either the need for a quick fix or in some cases, one simply loses their willpower to live.

Many of you are stuck in this vicious cycle, and it is a major crisis in the making. Serious trouble is ahead if this course does not change. This program will help you change course and break this vicious cycle.

Dangerous Definitions of Health

One of the main reasons people are not as healthy or thin as they could be is because our standard and accepted definition of health is completely wrong. Because of this, millions of you have been led to believe that you are much healthier, and safer from disease, than you truly are. Millions have died too young and millions have suffered needlessly. You have been told that conditions that are curable aren't. *Your power has been completely sucked away from you.*

The dangerous mistakes that are made regarding the definition of your health generally fall under one of three categories: You judge your health depending on how you look; you judge your health based on symptoms; and/or you judge your health based on blood tests. All three of these commonly used methods for determining your health are full of error and lead to much unneeded suffering, both in terms of your health and your weight.

How you look does not determine your level of health

When I was seriously ill, disabled, and unhealthy, I looked good. I was thin, tan, and attractive. I felt a bias from the doctors I saw because of this; that they judged my health based on my looks, and therefore discredited the seriousness of my condition. I don't think I was imagining this. I would love to see a study done in which this was measured; one where doctors where asked to determine one's level of health simply by looking at them. I am certain that this judgment is made all the time.

When someone is overweight and they complain of a symptom they are more likely to be taken seriously. Having doctors accuse me of being crazy was very stressful and difficult to endure. It also meant that it took a year and a half before any would agree to further testing, like an MRI, to determine what was going on. I kept asking about MRIs and CAT scans, but no one thought I needed one. If I were overweight would I have gotten the permission to do this sooner? (On the other hand, it eventually turned out to be a blessing that I was not taken seriously because had I been, I may have gone down the medical path, used drugs to treat my symptoms, and most likely, I would have been dead by now.) In the end, when the doctors finally agreed to do an MRI, I had become so disillusioned with the medical field and much more educated about alternative healing, that I knew I was going to take a different path. I knew that if I had this test done and it showed something scary like cancer, the fear might cripple me and prevent me from healing my body. So I never got that MRI after all.

I work in Boulder and see a lot of very active, fit and attractive clients who are extremely unhealthy. **Fit and healthy do not mean the same thing**. You look good when you are fit, but it does not mean that your organs and bowel are healthy. **How you look on the outside is not necessarily a reflection of how you look inside,** not if you are using exercise, a diet, plastic surgery, or any other crutch to manipulate your weight and looks.

Many fit, thin, and athletic people have died prematurely from cancer, heart disease, pneumonia, and other illnesses.

A recent article announced the following: "Overweight adults can be heart-healthy." Apparently this study revealed some "shocking" statistics. In measuring blood pressure, cholesterol, triglycerides, and blood sugar, it was found that 50% of overweight and 20% of obese people had normal levels of blood pressure, cholesterol, triglycerides and blood sugar and were considered to be in a healthy range, by medical standards. This is equivalent to approximately 56 million Americans. Additionally, the study revealed that about 25% of people who fall into a recommended weight range had at least two of the above variables that were unhealthy. This means some 16 million people, whom we consider safe from illness, are at risk of heart disease. I've been shouting this for a very long time!

Normal and healthy do not mean the same thing

Just because your doctor tells you your symptoms are normal does not mean you are as healthy as you could be. It is normal to be overweight and suffer with numerous symptoms in this country. It is normal to need some type of medication to make it through the day. So be careful when a doctor tells you your symptoms are normal, because "normal" is not where you want to be.

Symptoms do not necessarily reflect your level of health

Just because you may only have a few symptoms does not mean that you are as healthy as you could be, either. It is normal for a person who is diagnosed with cancer, or who has a heart attack to say, "But I had no symptoms that anything was wrong. I felt fine." In fact, heart disease is called the "silent killer" because so few symptoms precede death by heart attack. People drug themselves with medications, coffee, high protein diets, sugar, hours of exercise, and a lot of vitamins and are able to get through the day fine. But this does not mean that they are healthy.

On the other hand, I have worked with numerous clients who presented themselves to me with terrible, disabling symptoms, but a very healthy cellular system. In these cases, the high percentage of acids in their blood triggered numerous symptoms, but it also prevented the cellular damage that causes disease. They felt horrible, but they were free of cancer or heart disease, for example,

You cannot assume you are healthy because you have a relative few symptoms, and you do not need to assume you are near death's bed simply because you have many.

Our definition of normal is getting worse

Our definition of normal is gradually getting worse. Horrifically, as our health declines we seem to be accepting it. Why aren't we scared and concerned that more and more people are getting cancer at age forty than ever before? Will a large number of people have to start dying of heart disease and cancer at age thirty before we sit up and take notice, and demand that things change? Rather than ask, "How come asthma rates are so high now?" we just accept that having asthma is normal. It wasn't part of the "normal" definition ten years ago, so why is it now? A child today with asthma is considered healthy by medical standards, but they are not. As we get sicker, our new level of ill health is simply incorporated into our definition of health. This is extremely dangerous and needs to stop.

Not long ago, a doctor on television defended our current state of increased cases of A.D.D. in children simply as a result of a greater awareness of this condition and a greater likelihood of its diagnosis than in the past. There is some validity to this argument, but it also fraught with error. First of all, one conclusion we can reach about this is that we have been less healthy for longer than we thought! If kids with A.D.D. (a product of ill health), were in abundance yeas ago but simply not diagnosed, *then we're even worse off than we think*. We have been heading down the wrong road a long time. Second, there are many other conditions that are also associated with ill health that have been diagnosed for a long time that are on the rise, like diabetes. Since we have seen a consistent pattern of all conditions associated with ill health increasing, it makes sense that we truly have seen an increase in A.D.D. as well. Third, and most importantly, whether or not the cases have been increasing holds little relevance to what needs to be done to heal our bodies and those of our children. The past is the past. The future is the only thing we have control over. There is a great attraction to arguing that the medical approach is failing, and likewise, I understand the need that some doctors have to defend it. We need to let this go. Defending this position does nothing to help the future health and happiness of our children and ourselves. And our energy desperately needs to go towards healing the future right now.

We ignore symptoms that are relevant

It is said that 50% of the time, a heart attack is the first sign that anything is wrong. This statement is completely untrue. What the medical profession means is that often there's a lack of elevated blood cholesterol or shortness of breath, for example, prior to a heart attack. But there *are* symptoms that you are at risk—weight problems, depression, allergies, insomnia, skin problems, sugar cravings, gas, PMS, headaches, eczema, infertility, etc.; symptoms that reflect that your body is not as healthy as it could be and if left unchanged, will eventually turn into something worse, like heart disease.

When we accept symptoms like gas and PMS as normal, we are left shocked when something worse, like cancer, is diagnosed. **You need to respect, and react to, your health and weight problems *now*, before they become something deadlier.**

I have not had a pap smear in twenty years. This shocks many people, although I am at much lower risk of getting ovarian or uterine cancer than women who do. I am not simply waiting around for a diagnosis. Nor am I naïve, or in denial. I have taken my health into my own hands and am working to prevent cancer. I am not recommending that all of you women reading this do the same, although my female clients who do this program and regain their health are less likely to get these tests done. There is an educated and intuitive knowledge that they are safe from disease. I have periods every 28 days, they last only a few days, are light and comfortable, and I suffer zero symptoms of PMS. I do not take hormones or follow a diet or use any other crutch to accomplish this. This is the sign of a healthy hormonal body, one that doesn't get breast, ovarian, or uterine cancer. When I was younger and very unhealthy, my periods were seven days long, very heavy and uncomfortable, and I had symptoms of PMS. Then I was at risk for these cancers. If your hormonal symptoms are minor but you are taking hormones, this does not mean you are healthy. Or if you are on a high protein diet—you eat eggs, fish, chicken, or any other meat in total more than once a day—and you are free of symptoms, you are not necessarily healthy hormonally, either.

The main point of this discussion is to emphasize that when you are diagnosed with ovarian cancer, for example, you had many years of symptoms preceding this. You had warnings that "this" was coming, only everyone told you these symptoms were normal. So you did not respect them as warning signs. Wrongly, you were led to believe that you were in great health. Not only does this put you in a dangerously false place, but it makes you think that cancer, for example, "happens overnight." If you were "healthy" last year and got cancer the next, it must have occurred rapidly (which it absolutely does not), and surely this means there should be a "quick fix" to remedy it!

Just because you rarely get colds does not mean you are healthy

I often hear the comment; "I'm healthy because I hardly ever get sick." In most cases, "sick" is defined as getting colds or the flu. Meanwhile, the person making this comment may have had their gallbladder removed, suffers from PMS, has chronic back pain, or even cancer. But for some reason, they have come to define their health based on the number of times they get a cold or the flu. If someone has cancer, chronic back pain, or PMS, they are not healthy! *Do healthy people get colds? Yes. Is one's susceptibility to getting a cold an indication of that person's level of health? No.*

When I was sick with an autoimmune disease, I could barely make it through the day. I was in constant pain and discomfort. My nervous system was completely shot. During the three years that I was most disabled with my illness, I never once had a cold or flu. People would often say to me, "You can't be that sick, you never get sick." Since when have we come to define sick as getting colds, and not to include having diabetes, or any other immune disease? I have seen many clients who have a serious illness, like cancer or lupus for example, who explain how prior to their diagnosis they rarely got sick. I see a lot of clients who are very unhealthy and overweight, but who rarely get a cold.

When I began to heal my body and my debilitating symptoms went away, then and only then did I experience some colds. In fact, when I looked back at it, I never got "sick'" while in college, high school, and maybe even junior high school. I got sick when I was in elementary school. I remember those times, but I was considered "healthy" for many years after that. In truth, I was extremely unhealthy, as I was to find out a number of years later. When I suffered from colds again, I was becoming much healthier, not less healthy. My autoimmune disease was gone at this point. Many of my clients have had similar experiences.

Most of you have bought into the frequency of colds and flu as the determinant of your level of health, even though deep down, most of you have felt insecure about buying into this concept. You just didn't know how to define health differently, so you accepted this one. When I explain to a client the reason they never get a cold-- that their immune system is too weak to react to the cold virus by secreting mucus and creating the symptoms we associate with a cold, their faces light up with understanding and relief for finally getting an explanation of what they intuitively knew all along never made sense. Most importantly, it helps them understand and believe that maybe their migraines, for example, are not just genetic or stress-induced; maybe they are a product of less than optimum health. And because health can be improved, maybe their migraines can go away too…

A more accurate, although general, interpretation of your symptoms

In most cases, little kids are healthier than adults. Their symptoms, therefore, are reflective of healthier bodies. In general, "little kid symptoms" are a reflection of a healthier body than "adult symptoms." For example, if you only suffer from colds, allergies, ear aches, sore throats and/or acne—symptoms we see most frequently in younger children—you are much healthier than if you suffer from an autoimmune disease, osteoporosis, polyps, cyst, fibroids, plaque build-up in your arteries, diabetes, arthritis, hemorrhoids, colitis, and/ or Chron's disease, for example—symptoms that are seen more frequently in adults. When I help a client with acne, that person sees results much faster than the client who has hemorrhoids, because the acne client is much healthier, and has less work to do to heal their body in the first place. *Wrongly and dangerously, because many people with these more serious conditions do not also suffer from more obvious and sometimes more bothersome symptoms like acne or runny noses, they are labeled as healthy.*

The Problems with Blood and Other Tests

When your doctor checks your blood work and all of the variables that are measured, like calcium and glucose levels, are within the desirable range, he or she will conclude that you are in superb health and you will go on your merry way with a false sense of security, as well as a continued belief that all of your health and weight problems are unavoidable. You buy into the notion that it is simply your stressful job causing your eczema, or it is simply your lack of exercise that is causing your weight problems. You falsely and dangerously believe you are healthier and safer than you really are, and you walk out of the office continuing down the same ill-health producing path. I think it should be illegal for a doctor to pronounce you healthy only on the basis that your blood work comes back normal.

Normal blood work does not guarantee that you are in superb health. Many people with cancer, heart disease, and other significant illnesses have normal blood tests.

Of all the variables that must be kept within a delicate balance in your body in order for you to live, maintaining a balance, or homeostasis, of the variables in your blood is the most critical. Balanced blood chemistry is the number one priority of your body. And your body, the miraculous machine that it is, has numerous ways to make your blood normal if it becomes abnormal. *Except for your cholesterol levels,* if any of your blood components are out of balance, your body reacts appropriately to restore it. For example, there may not be enough calcium in your blood to help your heart contract and relax, which could be life threatening. In this case, your blood will borrow some from your bones. You need calcium in your bones, but it is more important that it is sufficiently present in your blood. *All of your organs and systems will sacrifice themselves for the sake of keeping your bloodstream in balance. Picture your blood as the king of the body and all of your other organs and systems as its servants.*

Your body's homeostatic mechanism is amazing but it also causes some significant problems. For one, it means that while your blood is taken care of, your organs become depleted. This can occur for a long time without you realizing that it is going on. In the above example, many years of calcium leaching out of your bones into your blood will lead to osteoporosis. Sixty to 70% of the calcium in your bones can be leached out before a low *blood* calcium level occurs. It is not until your bones become significantly depleted that they finally say to your blood, "Hey, I know you need our calcium but we are getting dangerously weak and we just can't give you much anymore." So your bones reduce the amount of calcium they give to your blood, and this finally becomes detectable in a blood test. How many women do you know who had normal calcium levels on their blood tests but a bone scan showed they have osteopenia or osteoporosis? If you start asking, you'll find that most women fall in this category.

Your blood cholesterol levels are not regulated by homeostasis. This means that if your levels become too high they stay too high; your body does not come to the rescue to lower them. Other organs are not harmed and depleted in an attempt to correct a high cholesterol level. The fact that cholesterol readings are included with all of the other ones on your lab results can lead to an even greater sense of false illusion about your state of health and power to change it. If your cholesterol readings are high but all of the other ones are within the desired range, you may be more likely to think that everything else in your body is perfectly normal. You may think, if one reading is out of range, surely others would be too if there was a problem. *If your blood cholesterol is high and your other blood variables are not, this does not mean that you are perfectly healthy and that your only "problem" is elevated cholesterol.*

The vast majority of our lives are spent in a state of sub-health, somewhere between optimum health and disease. States of sub-health do not appear on a blood test, yet these states indicate that there is a problem that can be changed. Dismissing the early warning signs, these troublesome symptoms that imply that things aren't exactly right in your body, spells more serious trouble later on. If these symptoms are blown off long enough, eventually your blood *will* show a problem, or you will have a heart attack or detect cancer. Finally you will get the support you need that your complaints warrant serious consideration. For some, this happens too late.

Do you know anyone who has shown up at their doctor's office a few months or a year after a complete blood work up in which everything was normal and they were told they were healthy, only to find they have cancer? This happens quite often, actually. Any oncology researcher will tell you that cancer takes decades to develop, not just months or a year. In other words, they were unhealthy and the cancer was there when the blood test was done, it simply wasn't detected. *You should never feel safe simply because your blood tests are normal.*

The above concepts detail what I believe are the gravest dangers of blood tests. There is one other, however; and that is the fact that it is estimated that anywhere from 30 to 50% of clinical tests are wrong. A study released in 2006 examined 120 clinical pathology labs where blood, urine, and other fluid tests are done, and estimated that each year in the United States, more than 2.9 million identification errors occur (when specimens are mislabeled or incorrect patient data is entered into a computer system). More than 160,000 patients are harmed in some way as a result, ranging from undue stress to death.

So why are so many blood tests done? They are cheap. And if a blood test did show that your liver was less than healthy, your doctors would not have an easy solution, i.e. drug, to prescribe to you for this anyway, so what incentive is there for them to demand better tests? In response to the question of why heart scans—a valuable test that measures the narrowing of your arteries and risk for heart attack—were not routinely prescribed, a *medical doctor* responded that this is because they do not have a drug to reverse this narrowing, but if they did, they would do these tests! *You deserve much better than this.*

What if my blood tests aren't all normal?

Sometimes a variable on your blood test will come back out of range and your doctor will tell you not to worry, it is no big deal. It is a big deal. Your body has to be relatively weak before an imbalance shows up. It may not be a disease or "cause for concern" from your doctor's viewpoint, but it can mean that you are closer to disease than if all of the components in your blood are normal.

If a variable is out of range on your blood work, it is advisable to re-test this in another couple of months or sooner, if your doctor recommends that you do so. Consistent readings that are out of balance are more significant than just one. *If you have abnormal tests they will change to normal as you heal your bowel and body.* As your bowel becomes healthier, it will be able to eliminate the acids that trigger homeostatic reactions from your organs that cause blood test variables to go up and down.

Other tests that lead you to crutches

When I was ill I went to many alternative health practitioners and took part in numerous testing methods, including muscle testing, hair analysis, live cell analysis, comprehensive metabolic and other blood tests, and pH tests done first thing in the morning and after eating. These tests also lead you to treat your symptoms and weight problems with crutches, and not heal your bowel and body.

Additionally, any time a doctor or alternative practitioner advises low carbohydrate, food allergy diets and/or the long-term ingestion of numerous supplements, you can be certain that their method of testing is a poor one and simply supportive of their attempt to treat your symptoms with crutches.

These tests have some value

Tests that have some value in determining the health of your body are: bone density tests and scans—like heart scans, MRIs, sonograms, body scans, mammograms, and biopsies. These tests reflect the health of your organs in a way that blood tests never can. There are fewer false negatives with these tests. A good blood test does not mean you are healthy; a bad blood test does not necessarily predict illness. A bad bone density test, on the other hand, means that your bones are unhealthy and a good bone density test means that your bones are healthy. These are relatively reliable tests. On the other hand, things have to get pretty bad before these tests show a problem, which *greatly limits* their value.

All of my clients do saliva and urine pH tests. I began studying about pH testing and using them with my clients over sixteen years ago, long before they became popular. You will find some articles and information on using them; unfortunately, they can be used two ways, and I only recommend one of them. When they are done the more common way, which is testing urine first thing in the morning or saliva right after eating, they lead to the application of more crutches.

While these tests are a wonderful tool for assessing your health, I will not be expanding upon them or explaining how to use them here. They are not necessary in order to heal your body, and the complexity of them would require many more pages of explanation of difficult concepts that I did not want to distract or confuse you with. I will attempt to tackle this in a future book.

Some of my clients do the other tests listed above as well. They are not required, but if desired or needed, they are recommended. Mostly, I do not recommend these as some of them can be expensive, and there is always the risk that they will evoke more fear than value for the individual.

Most of these tests are unnecessary

The majority of tests that your doctor or alternative practitioner has you do are much more beneficial to them then they are to you. And most of them are completely unnecessary.

Medical doctors love tests because they justify their approach to your health. They also support their recommendations for drugs and surgery. Remember the comment from the doctor about heart scans? This is entirely true for alternative practitioners as well. A test that shows you are low in a certain anti-oxidant, for example, makes it much easier for them to sell you some to take.

The following is an accurate definition of health that allows you to gage your level of health without the *necessity, expense, and unreliability* of a test.

An Accurate Definition of Health that You Can Feel Secure About

-- You have a complete lack of symptoms—no acne, gas, aches and pains, fatigue, insomnia, ongoing depression, PMS, high cholesterol, constipation, diarrhea, sugar cravings, etc.

-- You are thin and symptom-free, even if you are stressed or eating a lot of carbohydrates, wheat, or dairy products.

-- You have an abundance of energy without drinking caffeine in any form, or taking any other stimulant.

-- You feel great, without medications, vitamins, herbs, exercise, or chiropractic adjustments.

-- You have no addictions. Your body is not interested in sugar, alcohol, coffee, nicotine, or drugs.

-- Your bowel movements are twice a day and well-formed, even if you are stressed, or eat a lot of carbohydrates, spicy foods, raw vegetables, or dairy products. You do not have gas after eating beans or raw broccoli. If you are a woman, your stools do not get loose during your period.

-- You have no weight struggles. You don't have to diet or exercise to maintain it. You can eat a lot of carbohydrates and not gain weight. You do not have to constantly be vigilant about what you eat and how much you exercise. You are free of this "jail."

-- All of the medical tests that you do have—blood tests, pap smears, bone density tests, colonoscopies—show absolutely no abnormalities, not even non-cancerous polyps, cysts, ulcers, or any other items that you may be told are common and "nothing to worry about."

-- As a woman you do not suffer from symptoms of menopause or PMS. Your periods are every 28 days and you have no difficulty becoming pregnant and delivering your baby naturally. Your pregnancy and birth go smoothly and without complications.

-- It is effortless to maintain these results, and the results are long-term, meaning they last for decades.

-- You do not fear cancer or other diseases, because in great health, you do not feel insecure or vulnerable to them.

How many of you can answer "yes" to all of the above? The more "no's" you have, the more important it is for you to start healing your bowel and body now. If you have a lot of "no's," your health is not what it could be, regardless of what any other test has told you.

When you are done with this program you will pass this test. You will be able to answer "yes" to all of these questions. How many programs can deliver these kinds of results for you? Personally, this is the only one I am aware of that can.

Chapter Three

Why Healing Your Bowel Works

"When people understand things, they change their lives."
—Dr. Mehmet Oz.

I spend numerous hours educating my clients for the same reason: understanding your body and health is empowering. It helps you make the needed changes more easily than if I were to simply hand out a bunch of supplements and a diet to follow, as many health practitioners do. It may seem more complicated and time-consuming, but I do it because I know the process is much more effective as a result.

Understanding the physiology of pH balancing, and how your body's health breaks down, are necessary maps to get you on the right road and keep you there. "I believe that pH balancing is one of the keys to the future of medicine"—Dr. Elson M. Haas (*Delicious Living*, June 2007)

A healthy bowel eliminates the acids that trigger reactions from your body that lead to weight gain, illness, symptoms, addictions, and eventually, disease. Put another way, there are many dangerous consequences of *not* healing your bowel.

When you heal your bowel, you create a healthy bacterial environment within it. In addition to helping your body eliminate harmful acids, these bacteria plays key health and weight-regulating roles, and these are also discussed in this chapter.

It surprised me too!

When I first set out to heal my bowel and that of my clients, I knew this was a necessity for health, but I had no idea that this *alone* would result in the elimination of all symptoms, illness, addictions, and weight struggles, too. I had no idea how powerful this would be.

When I was ill I tried numerous programs and took thousands of herbs and supplements that I was led to believe would heal me. When none of these worked and I focused on my bowel, I experienced a complete and permanent elimination of all my symptoms. I knew that healing my bowel was the reason this happened, but I also figured that this was simply the missing link; that all of the other work I had done was healing my body but wasn't working because my bowel didn't work properly. I thought this other work was necessary for me to have achieved the miraculous results that I did. Only years later did I realize this was not the case. **This program will heal your bowel and body all by itself.**

I read hundreds of books and articles when I was ill and could find no information or studies done that described how healing the bowel alone could completely heal the rest of the body. I read books about how important the bowel was, but none that said that healing it alone could heal all of the other problems in the body, as all of these books also relied on crutches for the bowel like enemas, colonics, digestive enzymes, algae, etc.

When I first began my practice as a nutritionist I expected that my clients, too, would need to both heal their bowels and use a lot of other supplements for their other organs in order to fully improve their health. It was only after several years of working with clients, and finding that healing their bowel alone healed them of numerous health and weight problems, that I truly began to see the value and unlimited potential of this work. It also led me to focus even more aggressively on healing the bowel and to diminish my recommendations on other supplements and dietary restrictions.

Just How Important is Bowel Health?

It affects every health and weight symptom you have

The following is an old "story" about the bowel. It has relevance today and certainly in connection with the concepts of this program. It goes something like this: All the organs of the body were having a meeting, trying to decide who the one in charge was. "I should be in charge," said the brain, "because I run all the body's systems, so without me nothing would happen." "I should be in charge," said the blood, "because I circulate oxygen all over, so without me you'd waste away." "I should be in charge, "said the stomach, "because I process food and give all of you energy." "I should be in charge," said the legs, "because I carry the body wherever it needs to go." "I should be in charge," said the eyes, "because I allow the body to see where it goes." "I should be in charge," said the bowel, "because I'm responsible for waste removal." All the other body parts laughed at the bowel and insulted him, so in a huff, he shut down tight. Within a few days, the brain had a terrible headache, the stomach was bloated, the legs got wobbly, the eyes got watery and the blood was toxic. After that, they all decided that the bowel should be the boss.

Later in this chapter I describe the physiology of symptoms, weight gain, and disease and attempt to show you how and why the above story is true.

More support...

Seventy to eighty percent of your immune system is based in your bowel and fifty percent of your detoxification system. Your bowel contains 100 trillion microorganisms, which is ten times greater than the total number of cells in your body, and these are comprised of over 600 different species. If one considers this information alone, it appears as though our bowel was "chosen" to be the king of our body.

Your second brain

There are more nerve endings in your bowel than in your brain. Scientists have even called your bowel "your second brain." It is said that when your bowel is irritated, you will be too.

While many mental problems are the result of emotional stress, many others are the result of physiological stress. By healing your bowel, you heal your nervous system. Many of you will see this manifest as a reduction in depression, cravings, anxiety, irritability, and improved focus and mental capacity. By healing your bowel, you create an organ that can produce adequate amounts of brain chemicals that make you feel happy and good. When you treat your *physiological* mental and emotional problems with therapy only, failure is high as a result. When you heal your bowel and body, these issues are eliminated.

The research to support this

Dr. Lee M. Kaplan, MD, PhD, associate chief of the gastrointestinal unit at Massachusetts General Hospital says: *"If you have an unhealthy digestive system it's likely to make the rest of your body unhealthy as well."* When he mentions the digestive system, he is largely referring to your bowel. He is a unique doctor who recognizes and acknowledges the connection between the bowel and the health of the rest of your body. He has also been very involved in studying bowel health and you will see some references to his work throughout this book.

The relationship between bowel health and the impact of this on the health of the rest of the body is rarely studied. One of the few studies I could find was a 2003 study in the British Journal of Anesthesia found that 42% of constipated intensive care unit patients failed to be weaned from mechanical ventilation compared with 0% of the non-constipated patients. The median length of stay in the intensive care unit was 10.0 versus 6.5 days, respectively, and the proportion of the patients who failed to feed without an I.V. was 27.5% versus 12.5% respectively, in the constipated versus non-constipated patients. Not much of a study, huh?

It is not that the relationship between bowel health and the health of the rest of your body has been scientifically proven to not exist; it simply hasn't been studied.

Based on Science and Sensibility

The science of physiology explains how your body maintains homeostasis, or balance. You need to understand the basic scientific principles of human physiology before you can correctly interpret the information you read on health and nutrition, in here or elsewhere. Many other books fail to establish these principles, and *many definitely defy them.*

Ultimately, all of the information in this book ties back to the basic physiological and biochemical principles of the body, as we know them today. This program is based upon many years of personal research and experience, but it is equally based upon sound scientific principles. Explaining all of this in detail would be impossible, as well as complicated and boring. What follows is an explanation of the general concepts that are the most helpful to my clients in attaining success with this program.

It makes sense too

Understanding the science behind this is helpful, but is equally important that you trust your intuitive reaction that this information makes sense. This is especially true for my clients who have already had experiences with alternative health. If this is you, this will be much easier to grasp than if you are new to this arena, however, my intention is to explain things in a way so that *everyone* reading this can easily understand the principles, how and why it works, and how to make it work for them.

When I first learned about bowel health early in my illness I thought it made a lot of sense. I was ignorant about health and nutrition, yet the ideas presented in a little book about colon health stuck with me. For several years I gave myself over to the experienced professionals, and when they ignored the significance of my bowel health, I did too. I disregarded the information that had initially made sense to me, too. I trusted that these experts knew better. It was only after many horrific years of suffering and much expense that I returned to this information and the need to heal my bowel. As I began this process and finally experienced noticeable changes in my symptoms and health I often thought, "Wow, I can't believe I didn't trust my intuition…"

Trusting our intuition is difficult because of the fear that we will be wrong. But there is another way to approach this. First, ask yourself if you are acting out of what feels right or out of fear. *Fear and intuition are not the same.* Acting out of fear is not very helpful and can be harmful; acting out of intuition is much more valuable.

Second, keep in mind that there really are no wrong choices in life. For many years I traveled down the wrong roads searching for my health, but without these experiences, I never would have found the right one. Very few people are lucky enough to find the right road on their first try. My most successful clients are those who have also tried numerous approaches to their health and weight problems prior to seeing me. If you see every wrong turn as one step closer in the right direction, you too will be less fearful of making mistakes.

The Physiology of Healing

Did you know that your kidneys play an integral role in regulating your blood pressure? What would happen if every time someone was diagnosed with high blood pressure, they thought about what they could do to make their kidneys healthier? They might be less likely to turn to drugs, because have you ever heard about drugs being healthy for your kidneys? If you had kidney disease, even your doctor would advise a low animal protein diet. If you knew your kidneys were weak and contributing to your high blood pressure, would you be more likely to question the high protein argument? Maybe. Hopefully.

The less educated you are in human physiology, the more likely you are to fall for quick fixes that are harmful. The more likely you are to become confused, frustrated, and led down the wrong road. In most schools, biology and chemistry are core subjects, but physiology is not. I would love to see this change, but in the meantime, here is a brief course for you. If you are a nurse, chiropractor, or another health professional that has studied this topic more completely, read on as well. I have worked with a number of these individuals and they too appreciate and find value in the following. **Understanding how your body works minimizes fear and gives you power.**

Normal flow of acidity

One basic concept that will help you understand why this program works and how to heal your body is the general movement of acidity through your body. Every day your body is replacing some of its 100 trillion cells with new ones, and these old cells need to be discarded. You also have accumulated acids that were never eliminated, that your body continues to try to eliminate. Daily, you are also exposed to acidity through environmental chemicals and pollutants, your diet, and as a reaction to mental stress as well. If you breathe in pollution, for example, your body does not turn this into usable energy or material for building new cells, rather it is an unneeded waste product that must be eliminated.

Ideally, these accumulated acids and old cells, along with this new acidity, are sent into your bloodstream. From here, it should be sent into your lymphatic system and then into your bowel and other organs of elimination for excretion. Think of it like your house. The dirt you vacuum off the rug goes into a bag, this bag goes into a trashcan in your laundry room, and then this bag of trash goes into the large trashcan outside for the trash man to cart away. When all of these things happen, it helps your house stay clean.

This general flow chart will be useful to you as you read the remainder of this section. It is particularly invaluable when you read about high protein, low carbohydrate diets.

Maintaining pH Balance (Homeostasis)

In the last chapter I discussed how your body works to maintain homeostasis, or balance, when I discussed the problems with using blood tests to assess your health. I described how your body is constantly making homeostatic reactions, or adjustments, to keep your blood in balance, and how it will do this at the expense of the health of your organs. As a result of these adjustments, you will suffer from illness, symptoms, and overweight conditions. When you help your body correct the internal blood imbalances, you can dramatically improve the quality of your life. Miraculous healing can occur.

The most important component of your blood that needs to be kept in balance is the pH level. PH stands for "potential hydrogen." It is a measurement of relative acidity, as hydrogen ions are acidic. Alkalinity is at the opposite end of acidity. The range for pH is 0-14; 7 is neutral, 0 is the most acidic, and 14 is the most alkaline. The pH can be highly acidic, mildly acidic, mildly alkaline, or highly alkaline, for example.

If you garden or own a pool you know that the soil and pool water need to be maintained at a certain pH level. Your blood has an ideal pH level too, which is 7.4, or slightly alkaline. This pH needs to be maintained constantly. *Death occurs when it falls below 7.0.*

Your body is also busy correcting other imbalances in your blood, like blood sugar and calcium levels, but the pH level gets top priority. If your body could only correct one, and both the pH and calcium levels were out of balance, it would correct the pH level.

Your body has a lot of mechanisms to offset an overly acidic bloodstream. Thank goodness, because most of us are constantly acidifying it. Without all of these emergency repair mechanisms, most of us would have been dead a long time ago.

Your doctor will not routinely check your blood pH levels because they will always be at 7.4, unless you are in an accident and dying, or dying from a heart attack or other disease, at which point efforts in the emergency room or hospital will be directed towards stabilizing your pH. Likewise, it is insignificant to check these levels here as well.

What are significant to understand and measure are the effects that an unbalanced blood pH has had on your body over the course of many years. Every time your blood ph goes out of balance, your body immediately corrects this, but it does so at the expense of the rest of your body, and eventually health and weight problems surface. It is extraordinarily more common for your blood to become too acidic versus too alkaline, and henceforth I will refer only to this state of pH imbalance in this book.

What takes your blood pH out of balance?

Diet Everything that you eat is very acidic, slightly acidic, very alkaline, or slightly alkaline, and this affects your blood pH levels daily. The typical American diet is highly acidic. The popular high protein diets are especially acidic. The pH of food is scientifically measured and results primarily from the minerals that are contained in it. For example, potassium is a highly alkaline mineral and is found in large quantities in fruits and vegetables, which are alkaline-forming foods. Potassium and other alkalinizing minerals are not prevalent in foods like chicken, sugar, and white bread—all acid-forming foods. The digestibility of the food also affects its pH. Milk is a prime example. Although it contains large quantities of calcium, another alkaline mineral, it is very hard to digest, and undigested foods create acids. You have all heard that fruits and vegetables help prevent disease, and their alkalinity is a primary reason why. For more information on the ph of foods see Chapter 9.

Mental Stress Your blood pH becomes more acidic when you are stressed. You all know that "stress can kill," but few of you understand that it is the increased acidity in response to it that accounts for its harm to your health. Under stress your body produces a larger quantity of the hormone adrenaline to help you cope with it, and adrenaline has an acid chemistry. Also, deep breathing allows more acids to escape from your lungs than shallow breathing, and under stress we tend to take shallow breaths.

Environmental Stress And Chemicals Pollution, formaldehyde, pesticides, mercury, carbon monoxide, etc--all of these external chemicals affect the pH of your body and take it out of balance.

Drugs Prescription drugs and many recreational drugs are highly acidic.

The Sequence of Health Deterioration and Weight Problems

Understanding the process and order in which un-eliminated acids affect you is extremely important in order for you to understand how healing your bowel eliminates your symptoms, addictions, weight struggles and illness. It also provides a vital map that will help you understand the healing process and what to expect as you reverse the damage caused by these un-eliminated acids.

I talk about the body as though it were a long pipe. At the top of the pipe are your cells, bones and heart. In the middle are many of your digestive and blood-sugar regulating organs; and at the bottom are your lymphatic system and organs of elimination. Excess acids are handled in this order: first the bottom of the pipe, next the middle, and then the top.

The following is a description of the health and weight side effects of un-eliminated acids due to an unhealthy bowel. Put another way, none of the following reactions and subsequent symptoms would occur if your bowel were healthy.

The bottom of your pipe—your first line of defense against un-eliminated acids

When acids enter your body and into your blood, they should be sent into your lymphatic system and then down into your bowel for elimination.

Your other organs of elimination are your skin, kidneys, and lungs. These excrete acids via your breath, sweat, and urine. Your lymphatic system, which includes your spleen, thymus, and lymph nodes, does not eliminate acids directly, but rather carries them to your bowel to be eliminated (but I still include it in the "bottom of your pipe.")

These organs are your body's first line of defense against excess acidity. When you are exposed to excess acidity as a child, these are the first organs to respond to it. The bottom of your pipe clogs up first.

Every time these organs work hard to excrete acids, energy, enzymes, and nutrients are used, causing your elimination organs to become weaker.

As your bowel responds to un-eliminated acids this produces symptoms of *bloating, gas, constipation, diarrhea, fissures, hernias, bacterial and yeast infections, hemorrhoids, diverticulitis, Chron's disease, appendicitis, I.B.S., or colitis,* for example.

When your kidneys respond to un-eliminated acids this affects your water balance regulation, and regulation of your blood pressure and circulation. After many years of stress to your kidneys you may experience *water retention and weight gain, edema, high blood pressure, and/or cold hands and feet,* for example. Other reactions include: *acne, bladder infections, cystitis, dehydration, difficulty holding urine, hot flashes, kidney infections, low energy, low sex drive, mental fogginess, nighttime urination or frequent daytime urination, or poor memory.*

As your lungs respond to un-eliminated acids you may experience *asthma, allergies, coughs, or bouts with pneumonia, bronchitis, or emphysema.*

As your skin responds to these un-eliminated acids you may experience *acne, hives, boils, eczema, rashes, psoriasis, dry skin, oily skin, or dandruff.*

Your lymphatic system responds to un-eliminated acids by secreting inflammatory chemicals to buffer them, resulting in *pain and inflammation,* like *headaches, neck pain, back pain, arthritis and other "itis" conditions.* Additional symptoms include *allergies, anemia, anxiety, autoimmune diseases like lupus, fibromyalgia, and chronic fatigue; breast pain and lumps, colds, dizziness, earaches, fibroids, headaches, herpes, miscarriages, sore throats, neck pain, prostate problems, ringing in your ears, TMJ, and thyroid, or TSH, imbalances,* for example.

Depending on your genetic inheritance and the nature of the toxin/acid you are exposed to, these organs of elimination usually weaken at the same time. In other words, few people have weak kidneys and yet strong lungs, skin, and bowels. When I was younger, I had constipation, appendicitis, profuse sweating, and frequent kidney infections, which are signs of bowel, skin, and kidney weakness.

Think of the common childhood illnesses and you will notice that many of them are symptoms of your body trying to eliminate excess acids. For most young people, their body is still strong enough to be actively "using" this first line of defense to keep itself in balance. For example, one can experience diarrhea, constipation, stomachaches (bowel weakness); congestion and running noses (lymphatic weakness); acne, eczema, and rashes (skin weakness); bedwetting (kidney weakness); and asthma (lung weakness). These symptoms are much more common in children than those associated with weaknesses in your body's second and third lines of defense, like diabetes, high cholesterol, osteoporosis, and heart disease.

Your body is truly amazing, as it chooses these organs as its first line of defense against excess acidity. Depleting these organs is much safer than depleting your other ones. It is statistically safer to get skin cancer than it is to get pancreatic cancer, for example. Your organs of elimination are the first to weaken, and they are also the "safest" ones to become unhealthy, as well.

You are not healthy if you outgrow asthma, or any other childhood symptom

Unfortunately we spend a lot of time, money, and energy trying to stop these primary elimination symptoms. In fact, while these symptoms are the least dangerous, they are usually the most annoying and bothersome. They are the ones that clients want to get rid of most of all. Forcing your body to eliminate these symptoms is undesirable, however. If you use a drug to make your acne go away, for example, then you may block your skin as an organ of elimination, and this means that your body must find another way to deal with the un-eliminated acids that are causing the acne in the first place. It may use some of the nutrients from your liver to handle these acids, for example, and an unhealthy liver is much more dangerous than unhealthy skin. I am not suggesting that you learn to live with acne if you have it. I am suggesting that forcing your body to eliminate a symptom can be harmful to the rest of your health. The best way to eliminate a symptom, healthfully and permanently, is to heal your bowel.

Additionally, many of you have wrongly and harmfully been led to believe that you are healthier when your childhood symptoms "disappear." A common medical approach is to avoid them. Doctors often tell you that they will most likely stop occurring eventually on their own. People always think this means that they magically went away and they are now healthier. Take asthma, for example. Children often "outgrow" this condition. When you "outgrow" a condition—and have not healed your body, but simply went along with life and waited for it to disappear—what really happened is your organs of elimination became too unhealthy to completely offset all of the un-eliminated acids, and your other organs are now responding to them. Your asthma will be replaced with another problem, and this should not be interpreted as good. When I was young I had a lot of strep throat that I "outgrew" too. However, since these symptoms were ignored and nothing was done to help the health of my body, I eventually "grew into" an autoimmune disease! The sore throats were gone, but I was half dead. Great trade off, huh?

The middle of your pipe—your second line of defense

After your organs of elimination have weakened, and as un-eliminated acids continue to occur and accumulate, your body eventually turns to its *second line of defense: your liver, gallbladder, pancreas, stomach, small intestine, and adrenal glands* to offset the potential harm and death caused by them. As I say, the trash begins to build up in the middle of your pipe.

These organs react to un-eliminated acids to protect you as well, but their reactions are different from those of your organs of elimination. For example, your liver makes more cholesterol and fat to entrap these acids, which manifests as *elevated blood cholesterol levels and weight gain.* Additional problems that occur at this level are *low blood sugar (craving sweets, alcohol and /or nicotine), diabetes, depression, gastritis and reflux, hormonal imbalances and infertility, hepatitis, fatigue, and a lowered metabolism,* to name a few.

It is more dangerous for these organs to weaken than it is for your elimination ones, but it is less dangerous to have these weaken than it is for the following.

The top of your pipe—your third line of defense

The same process eventually occurs whereby these organs become too unhealthy to buffer the un-eliminated acids and keep your blood pH in balance, at which point your third line of defense is utilized to do this. *This includes the bone and cells of your body.*

At this point, your body uses up calcium and magnesium from your bones, as these are highly alkaline minerals that can be used to neutralize, or buffer, the un-eliminated acids in your blood. Your bones contain a lot of calcium and magnesium, although eventually the supply will run low and you will end up with *osteoporosis*, a life-threatening disease.

Your body will also steal some sodium and potassium from your intra- and extra- cellular fluids. Sodium and potassium are also highly alkaline minerals, and these too can be used to neutralize the un-eliminated acids in your blood. This process will eventually cause life-threatening harm, as these minerals are needed by your cells to maintain their health and prevent *degeneration, like arthritis and cancer.* When your cells die, you do too. At this level, you are at risk of *stroke* and *heart disease,* as cholesterol and plaque accumulate on your arterial walls. A lowered metabolism, due to thyroid insufficiency, will lead to more *weight gain* as well as greater bouts of *fatigue and mental disorders.*

Once the un-eliminated acids "reach the top of your pipe" you are in big trouble. It is life threatening.

In 2004, researchers at Harvard Medical School and Hebrew Rehabilitation Center for Aged found that women with thin hand bones were 27% more likely to develop heart disease than those who had the sturdiest bones. Your heart and bones weaken at the same time, although not at the same rate. A heart scan, which shows the accumulations of plaque on the arterial walls, can therefore not only help predict risk of heart disease, but your risk of dying from another degenerative disease as well, as arterial accumulations and cellular death occur concurrently. Likewise, a bone scan not only can predict the onset or occurrence of osteoporosis, but if this is found, you should also be concerned about the health of your heart and cells as well.

A gradual process of deteriorating health

In summary, every organ in your body has a unique ability to protect you from un-eliminated acids, and these responses lead to symptoms, weight gain, and disease. As time goes by, acids accumulate in your body and move towards the "top of your pipe."

Not all of the above symptoms will occur at the same time. For example, your lymphatic system (often referred to as your immune system) initially reacts to these acids by entrapping them with mucus secretions, which results in congestion, runny nose, and other symptoms of a cold. As your lymph system becomes weaker, it turns to more aggressive ways of dealing with these acids, such as secreting compounds into your lymph fluid to neutralize them, producing pain and inflammation. If you experience arthritis, for example, but never gets colds, it means that your lymphatic system is indeed weak, and in fact weaker than if you got colds but had no arthritic pain.

From the above description of how your body breaks down you can see why so many of us can get away with a very poor diet or excess stress before paying the price. I thought I was getting away with murder all of the years that I abused drugs and alcohol and ate horrendously. Likewise, many of you eat whatever you want as children and teens and yet are still able to maintain your weight very easily. You are told that if you are thin you don't need to worry about what you eat. But you do! If you eat poorly as a youngster, your organs of elimination will weaken, and one day you will have a struggle on your hands. Often, your excess weight or health problem seems to "appear out of nowhere," but this is entirely untrue. All health and weight problems are the result of a great accumulation of un-eliminated acids in your body, coupled with an unhealthy bowel bacterial environment. If you struggled with these problems when you were very young, you unfortunately inherited a very unhealthy bowel, and you have a much greater chance of struggling with more serious issues at a relatively young age, like cancer at age forty.

Whether your condition has developed "overnight" or has been around a long time, you must realize that it takes a lot of time before these un-eliminated acids accumulate to the degree that they cause great discomfort or alarm, and it will take time to reverse this. There is no possibility of a magic pill or quick fix to do this. You buy into these constantly, but if you understood the physiology of how your body works, maybe you would stop wasting your time and money going down these wrong roads.

Most importantly, if your body is healthy and can eliminate the acids from diet, stress, drugs, chemicals and pollutants, these don't have much of a damaging effect on your body. It is not the rain that ruins your house but the holes in the roof that allow the rain to get in. This is why one hundred people can all be exposed to the same carcinogenic chemical and yet only eight may develop cancer, for example. If the chemical were the cause of the cancer, then all one hundred individuals would get cancer, but this is not what we see.

A Healthy Bowel Reverses This Process

In this program, this degenerative process is reversed when your bowel is healed. As your bowel becomes healthier, only then can your body eliminate the accumulation of acidity that is weakening your other organs. The trash in your house can only get out when there is space in your trashcan.

You cannot remove the trash that is in the middle of your "pipe" if the bottom is clogged. The trash that is in the middle of your pipe cannot come out the sides of your pipe; it must exit below, where your bowel and other organs of elimination channels are. Of these, your bowel is the most important. Think of it as the large trashcan that you place outside, and think of your kidney, skin, and lung trashcans as the small trashcans in your bathroom, kitchen, etc. They are important, but your bowel is significantly more so.

When excess acidity is eliminated, your organs become nourished and heal. The symptoms that you started with disappear. The majority of other alternative health programs require a large intake of vitamins and herbs that help replenish the nutrients lost by an acidic body, but they do nothing to eliminate the acids that are causing the depletion in the first place. This eventually leads to failure and only short-term and minimal improvements in your health and weight, as well as a susceptibility to premature disease. *Also, these vitamins do not stop the continued accumulated of acids in your body.*

I have never worked with an overweight client, or one with symptoms, addictions, illness, or disease, who has come to me with a healthy bowel, and I have never seen a client improve the health of their bowel and not see a remarkable improvement in their health and weight.

Additional Effects of Un-Eliminated Acids Due to an Unhealthy Bowel

The pH of your blood regulates significant metabolic processes necessary for life. For example, it regulates breathing and energy production within your cells. It regulates oxygenation of your blood, and without sufficient oxygen you would die. Body electricity is also controlled by pH. Without this electrical current you would die.

By helping your body eliminate acids, a healthy bowel improves circulation, hydration, oxygenation, and nutrient levels in your body.

Your body buffers un-eliminated acids with oxygen, and a decrease in oxygenation results in slow healing times, bacterial infections, Candida, low energy, anemia, lung problems like asthma, lowered brain function, "brain fog," stroke, and cancer.

Excess acids further decrease the beneficial bacteria in your bowel, resulting in bacterial infections, immune disorders, Candida, vaginal infections, thrush, low energy, food allergies, difficulty sleeping, breast and prostate cancer, cysts, tumors, and fibroids. The bacterial functions are discussed in greater detail later in this chapter.

Excess un-eliminated acids cause a decrease in the production of hydrochloric acid, resulting in ulcers, stomach pain, food allergies, inflammation, and difficulty gaining muscle weight.

They also cause a decrease in the production of digestive enzymes resulting in weight gain, allergies, diabetes, hypoglycemia, bloating, and gas.

Excess acidity reduces circulation, which impedes healing, results in cold hands and feet, and an increase in aches and pains.

Excess acidity disturbs the secretions of insulin, adrenaline, and thyroxin. It reduces the assimilation of fat soluble vitamins—A, D, E, and K—which need a correct pH in bile and pancreatic juices to be assimilated by your body, and triggers a reaction from your nervous system which responds to these acids—irritating it, and you, and reducing neurotransmitter production—which affects yours brain and can trigger anxiety, depression, sugar cravings and other addictions.

Dangerous bacteria and cancer thrive in an acidic blood environment, which exists when your bowel is unhealthy.

In *This Works, Crutches Don't 2*, I provide more detailed descriptions of a select number of health conditions and further show you the connection between these and a healthy bowel.

pH Fears, Misunderstandings, and Other Important pH Concepts

pH fears on the Internet

Several years ago I was directed to an article on the Internet regarding pH and cancer. The article was titled "Calcium Doesn't Cure Cancer: The Real Story About pH and Cancer." I believe this originated in to defense to the popular and successful infomercials on television at the time selling coral calcium. The infomercials claimed that calcium, an alkaline mineral that improves your pH, could cure cancer.

Most people who read this article would be confused and likely sold on the idea that calcium is of no value, potentially harmful, and that this pH stuff is all rubbish. And while I agree that taking calcium would be insufficient to cure cancer, as it is a crutch and crutches don't cure you, there is great value in using calcium as a short-term crutch. More importantly, there is great need to properly understand the science of pH, as it is the foundation of healing.

The article was clever and very misleading. It was very long and my response could be much longer, showing you the ignorance of the information stated, but I will restrict myself to addressing the key mistakes in it. They were repeated numerous times. The average person reading his article may have judged the author's knowledge and arguments as substantial, but as I will show you, they all stem from the same misunderstandings about pH and health. The better you understand this, the more empowered you will be to heal your body.

Ideal pHs of your organs and other measurements

To fully understand the invalidity of this article you must first know that there are different ideal pH values depending on which pH you are referring to. *Your blood pH should be 7.4, but this is not the ideal pH of your organs.* The approximate ideal pH values of the following organs are: small intestine, 8.0; stomach, 2.0; pancreas, 9.5; bladder, 8.5; large intestine, 6.0; prostrate, 5.5. This is a measurement of the pH of their mucous membranes and secretions. For example, your stomach ideally has a low, highly acid pH because it also produces hydrochloric *acid* to help you digest your food. Some organs need to be acidic and others need to be alkaline in order to be healthy. *When your blood is acidic, because your bowel is not eliminating acids, these other ideal pH's are disturbed as well.*

Calcium alkalinizes your *blood*

Calcium, along with magnesium, potassium, and sodium, is an alkalinizing mineral that helps keep your <u>blood</u> *from becoming too acidic.* When your *blood* is too acidic, the health of the rest of your body suffers, as described earlier.

Throughout this article, however, the author referred to various situations where the administration of an alkalinizing agent to an *organ,* like the bladder, has resulted in higher incidences of cancer in that organ. Because of this, he wrongly and dangerously concluded that an alkalinizing agent, like calcium, not only does not cure cancer, but also can cause higher incidences of it.

Calcium alkalinizes your blood. Calcium does <u>not</u> *alkalinize your organs.* In order for your organs to be of the optimum, healthy pH, your blood pH cannot be overly acidic. *By buffering acids in your blood, calcium helps create the ideal pH level in your organs.*

Here is a significant paragraph copied from "Human Physiology" by Vander, Sherman and Luciano. In referring to ulcers it states on page 546: *"Many patients with ulcers have normal or even subnormal rates of acid secretion."* No more is said about this significant finding, because they don't know what to make of it. Alkalinizing your blood helps acidify your stomach and bowel. Some foods and supplements, like hydrochloric acid, acidify your stomach and bowel, and are valuable because of this.

Time again I see clients who are confused about this process because someone else has discussed pH's with them but failed to clarify *which* pH they were referring to. The blood? Bladder? Stomach? Or saliva? *A lot of pH theory is discredited as a result of this oversight.*

The author brought up other examples where an alkaline organ is unhealthy and he is right. **But to imply that ingesting calcium will alkalinize an organ is 100% wrong.**

He also mentions that there is excessive calcium in tumor cells. Yes that is true, but it is not the result of taking calcium supplements. It is, rather, an attempt by your body to protect itself. This wrong and dangerous correlation is made in other cases as well, and you will find this discussed again later in this book.

The presence of a nutrient does not mean it caused the problem. If firemen show up at your burning house to put out the fire, don't blame them for starting it simply because they are there! Rather, their presence at the fire is an attempt to protect your house.

Someone I know was diagnosed with incurable cancer of his blood. A couple years prior to this diagnosis, he began to complain about itchy bumps on his skin. He had numerous medical tests done to try to determine the cause, but nothing was found. They even looked for cancer at this time. Bone density tests were not performed. Later on I saw him in person and immediately recognized the bumps as calcium deposits. I suggested that he start talking extra calcium supplements because I knew this was a very dangerous situation. I knew that calcium was leaching out of his bones to protect his acidic blood; that his body and cells were degenerating rapidly, and that he would never be able to accept any other knowledge I could share with him about healing his body. The calcium supplements were meant to help minimize the depletion of calcium from his bones into his blood to buffer the acidity there, thus minimizing the formation of the calcium deposits that were popping out of his skin. I knew that these deposits were an extreme, urgent, last-chance, "top of the pipe" effort by his body to keep his blood pH in balance. He began taking the extra calcium.

Shortly after my visit he was diagnosed with cancer, as I predicted, and the medical profession finally did a bone density test and guess what they found? Sure enough, as I had discovered by looking at his skin, his bones were severely depleted of calcium and dangerously weak.

It was also found that he had high blood levels of calcium, a situation that occurs when large amounts of calcium are exiting your bones to buffer the acids in your blood. Remember the bone density test confirmed the depletion of calcium in them. He told the doctor that I had advised the calcium supplements and the doctor told him to stop taking them because they could be harmful given his high blood levels of it. He stopped, but this did not result in a reduction of his high blood calcium levels. The reason his blood levels were high was because his body was very unhealthy and was dumping calcium into his blood to help protect him from a very large quantity of un-eliminated acids. **Taking calcium supplements does not cause high blood levels of calcium (on the contrary!),** and I dare anyone to find a single study that proves to the contrary. The doctor's advice for him to stop the supplements was based on ego, fear, and/or ignorance. It was not in the best interest of the health of his patient, who recently died after a long, debilitating battle with this cancer.

It's mostly about pH

Numerous studies—way too many to count and list here—have found that the consumption of alkalinizing foods, like fruits, vegetables, and tea, reduce ones incidence of death from disease. Unfortunately, the alkalinity of these foods never gets any credit for these results; rather, some other explanation is theorized, such as a higher level of anti-oxidants or fiber contained in some of these foods. On the flip side, numerous studies—way too many to count—have found that the consumption of foods like sugar, alcohol, refined salt, chicken, beef, turkey, and hydrogenated fats reduce health and longevity. These foods are highly acidic.

Likewise, numerous studies—too many to count—have found that alkalinizing minerals like calcium dramatically reduce one's incidence and death from disease. For example, a recent six-year study involving 73,000 women out of Vanderbilt University, National Cancer Institute, and Shanghai Cancer Institute, found that women who had the highest intake of calcium reduced their colorectal cancer risk by 40%, compared to women with the lowest intake. That is a significant, credible study.

In my office calcium supplements are used as a short-term crutch. There is a much more effective and complete way to prevent your organs from becoming too alkaline, and you from developing stones or tumors. In the end, a healthy bowel will do a much better job of keeping your blood alkaline and the pH of your organs healthy than calcium supplements. If your healthy bowel eliminated all of the extra acids in the first place, there would be no need for extra calcium. Calcium will not fix your bowel.

Saliva and urine pH testing

I conduct urine and saliva pH tests with my clients. These measure the relative amount of acidity and ill health in their body and reflect which organs this has affected. They show "how far up the pipe" the trash has gone. For example, I can tell if the immune system is depleted as well as the cellular system, which makes one more susceptible to cancer, or if just the immune system is weak. These tests are individually assessed and difficult to explain and interpret here. I mention it, however, because there is also a lot of confusion about pH testing, and I want to mention it briefly in case you have ever tested yours. I have done pH testing with every client I have seen in the last fifteen years and am very knowledgeable about them. The worse your pHs are, the more dangerous this is. On the other hand, *perfect pHs are great, but they alone do not mean perfect health. Your pH's can be good if your bowel is very unhealthy, and an unhealthy bowel, by itself, will create health and weight problems, as the following description will show you.*

Functions of Healthy Bowel Bacteria

Your bowel is home to approximately 100 trillion bacteria, and at any time your bowel will contain some bad, or harmful, bacteria, as well as viruses, Candida, yeast, and fungi. Some of the names of the harmful bacteria are staphylococcus, streptococcus, salmonella, clostridium, and Escherichia. The majority of the bacteria in your bowel, however, should be good, beneficial ones. Some of these are called L.acidophilus, L. bifidus, L.rhamnosus, B.lactis, and S.boulardii, for example. Some of the terms you will see that are used to describe the bowel bacteria are: beneficial bacteria, flora, cultures, and acidophilus.

For many reasons, *especially genetic*, this balance is upset in most of you. When there are insufficient numbers of beneficial bacteria in your bowel, many of its functions cannot be performed sufficiently.

It is not enough to eliminate acids

In addition to the numerous benefits you will receive by healing your bowel and eliminating excess acids as described earlier, a healthy bowel bacterial environment directly improves your health and weight in other ways as well. This is why *it is not enough to simply fast or do other things to eliminate acids.* This is very beneficial, but it is incomplete and non-permanent. **If you don't heal your bowel you'll need crutches forever to stay thin and healthy. No one can use crutches forever! If you eliminate all of the old acids from your body but do not heal your bowel bacterial environment, you are still at risk of ill health and disease.**

You need to both get all of the grime out of your house and fix the holes in the trashcan that allowed it to accumulate in the first place. When you heal the intestinal bacteria, you fix the holes.

Some of the primary functions of your healthy intestinal bacteria are discussed below.

Formation of acids into stools that can be quickly and efficiently eliminated

Infrequent and/or poorly formed stools can be the result of poor intestinal bacteria. Ultimately this directly leads to the re-absorption of acids, which cause weight problems, illness, symptoms and disease, as described earlier in this chapter. Indirectly, this supports your health because it is only when your bowel is healthy that you will feel comfortable and not gain weight when you eat a healthy, healing, low protein, high fiber diet. *Most supplements, diets, and physical modalities do not eliminate acids; a healthy bowel does.*

Holes in the trashcan, or leaky gut syndrome

What I call "holes in the trash can" is more commonly referred to elsewhere as a condition called leaky gut syndrome. They are the same thing. The leaky gut educators describe this condition the following way: "A healthy intestinal lining allows nutrients to enter the body uninhibited, while preventing toxins within the digestive system from being absorbed into the bloodstream and producing adverse reactions elsewhere in the body. When the digestive lining becomes inflamed, these functions become compromised. The lining becomes hyper permeable and permits toxins and other undigested food particles, especially large protein molecules, to be absorbed into the bloodstream, subsequently causing allergic reactions and inflammation elsewhere in the body."

In my practice it is explained that your bowel bacteria turn acids into stools, which then carry these acids out of your body, preventing them from becoming reabsorbed and triggering health, weight, and disease conditions.

"Leaky gut" is a condition that is eliminated by healing your bowel bacteria. Once I had a client leave my program early because another practitioner diagnosed her with this condition, and she thought it was different from what we were doing. There may be other names for this condition that I am not aware of, so if you come across any do not be misled or confused. An unhealthy bowel is an unhealthy bowel, no matter how you describe it.

The truth is, a healthy gut *is* porous and has "holes" in it that can "leak." It is just when the acids in it are not formed into a stool—because the intestinal bacteria are not strong enough to do this—that the acids become re-absorbed. Only the unformed acids get reabsorbed, not the formed ones. In other words, I do not agree that the "leaky gut" is causes the re-absorption of acids. If all of the acids in your bowel were efficiently formed into a stool by your bowel bacteria, no acids would be re-absorbed, holes or not. Likewise, when I use the term "holes in your trashcan" it is not to be taken literally, either. It is simply meant as an analogy to help you understand how to heal your bowel and body.

Digestion of insoluble fiber

Your bowel bacteria help with the digestion of insoluble fiber from foods like corn, beans, lettuce and other raw vegetables, whole grains, and seeds, and results in *greatly reduced gas when eating these foods, better formed stools, an absence of undigested food in your stool, and less bloating.* When the bowel bacteria are unhealthy, people tend to avoid these healthy foods because of the discomfort caused by eating them. Eating disorders are prevalent when food consumption causes discomfort and bloating. All of the clients I have ever worked with who have anorexia or bulimia have extremely weak bacterial environments in their bowel.

The benefits of a high fiber diet on your health and weight have been studied and proven numerous times. Fiber also increases insulin sensitivity and supplies IP6, which tames cancer cells, sometimes making them disappear. Fiber is filling, and people who eat it often crave less food. High fiber foods also lower cholesterol levels. It is said that the beneficial bowel bacteria in your bowel ferments fiber into short chain fatty acids, which then turn down the action of your body's enzyme HMG COA reductase, thereby suppressing cholesterol synthesis in your body. (Short-chain fatty acids are also used to help heal the bowel. If your bowel bacteria are weak, this process will not occur.) My description is that fiber helps "move" the acids out of your blood into your bowel, reducing the production of cholesterol that occurs as your body attempts to buffer these acids.

High fiber foods are very healthy and a healthy bowel will encourage the consumption of them in your diet.

Hormonal regulation

Women make estrogen in their ovaries, a few other organs, and body fat. Estrogen flows through your body one time, stimulating your breasts, uterus, ovaries, and skin. After one passage through your bloodstream it goes to your liver, where it is attached to another substance and conjugated, or "bound." Conjugated estrogen, which is not absorbable, is excreted into your bowel to be eliminated through your stools.

Unfriendly bacteria deconjugate estrogen, or free it up, and allow it to pass through the body again, contributing to disease. Excess re-absorption of estrogen is implicated in the majority of ovarian, uterine, and breast cancers, endometriosis, fibroids, cysts, infertility, and PMS. A healthy bacterial environment allows this unwanted estrogen to be eliminated, preventing these conditions and diseases.

In 2002, studies estimated that up to 40% of women 35 and older already have or will develop uterine fibroids. These can cause excessive bleeding and pain, as well as lead to infertility or cancer. And unregulated hormones interfere with a woman's ability to have a successful pregnancy without miscarriage.

Your intestinal bacteria play a key role in regulating the production and balance of male hormones too. As with estrogen, testosterone is a hormone that helps stimulate the male organs and creates health, but an excess of testosterone can also be harmful. Like estrogen, *a healthy bacterial environment in the bowel is necessary to prevent the excessive re-accumulation of testosterone into your body. Excess levels of testosterone have been implicated in prostate cancer, low sperm counts, reduced sex drive, and an inability to sustain an erection.*

Manufacture of vitamin B-12

Poor intestinal bacterial health causes low levels of vitamin B-12 production. *Low levels of B-12 have been implicated in cases of depression, low energy, and nerve damage.* It is also needed to prevent anemia.

Vitamin B-12 is needed for the production of the neurotransmitter serotonin and benzodiazepines. Valium and Xanax are pharmaceutical benzodiazepines. Recently an article appeared in the *New York Times* touting the benefits of vitamin B-12 for depression.

Without enough B-12, your body does not formulate enough SAMe (S-adenosylmethionine), an important mood regulator that boosts serotonin levels in your brain. Also, studies show that up to 30% of people hospitalized for depression have low blood levels of B-12. A study published in the December 2003 issue of *BioMed Central Psychiatry* found that after six months of studying 115 Finnish patients with major depressive disorder, those who experienced a greater than 50% reduction in symptoms had the highest blood levels of vitamin B-12.

When there is insufficient B-12, the sheath surrounding the delicate nerves of your brain and spine suffer. Nerve damage is most notable in some autoimmune diseases such as multiple sclerosis, Lou Gehrig's disease, Alzheimer's and Parkinson's, as well as in other nervous system/brain disorders such as autism, ADD, and seizures.

Vitamin B-12 is involved in the conversion of homocysteine into methionine, and lower homocysteine levels are implicated in lower levels of heart disease and stroke, as was found in a 2005 study that followed 559 elderly stroke patients. *People who tend to have higher homocysteine levels are 2-4 times more likely to suffer hip fractures.* In a two-year study, half of the participants took 5 mg of folic acid and 1,500 mcg of vitamin B-12, and the others took a placebo. Even though both groups sustained roughly the same number of falls during that time, the treatment group suffered 80 percent fewer fractures. (It is unknown how exactly these two nutrients help bone health.) They also saw their homocysteine levels drop, whereas the patients taking the placebo saw their levels increase.

Vegan diets have long been criticized as lacking in sufficient vitamin B-12, as it is found in meat and dairy products, which vegans do not eat. A healthy bowel will produce sufficient amounts of B-12 for you, and a vegan diet—which is low in acidity, easy to digest, and high in fiber—helps create a healthy bowel, although *a vegan diet by itself does not guarantee a healthy bowel bacterial environment.* Ironically, a meat-based diet, which is high in B-12, is also very harmful to your bowel, and many of my clients who have seen improvements by taking B-12 eat more animal protein than they should. Vitamin B-12 deficiencies are a product of an unhealthy bowel, not of a low-animal protein diet. A new vegan may have a very unhealthy bowel when they begin eating this way and may be found to be deficient in B-12, but this is not due to their diet; rather, the blame lay in their lack of bowel health.

Twenty years ago when I was very ill, I received weekly B-12 shots. The amount I was given was inadequate to produce results, and because no one knew how to heal my bowel, the results I received from these were minimal and very short-lived. I recommend supplements of vitamin B-12 as a crutch, and find these to be more effective than shots because they can be taken more consistently and for longer periods of time if needed. Not many people will get a shot five days a week for months on end.

I have seen significant reductions in clients' pharmaceutical and recreational drug, alcohol, coffee, and sugar cravings and usage with the addition of sufficient amounts of vitamin B-12, as well as noticeable improvements in neurological symptoms in adults and kids with autism, A.D.D., and similar disorders. For more information on using this crutch while you heal your bowel, see Chapter 10.

Absorption of calcium

Calcium has to be ionized in your intestines in order to be absorbed, and your bowel bacteria play a key role in this, resulting in an improvement in your bone health. Studies have shown that calcium is more readily absorbed in the presence of fermented lactic cultures, such as yogurt. (Fermented diary products are easier to digest than ones that are not, making the calcium within them more available to your body. *Absorption* of calcium is critical for bone health). Just the other day a client brought in an article in the newspaper that claimed that the "answer" to preventing osteoporosis might lie in the bowel!

Calcium mal-absorption is a significant cause of bone loss, osteopenia, and osteoporosis. Taking in more calcium, via the diet or supplements, does not always prove beneficial to your bones because the calcium does not always get absorbed effectively. Also, remember that if acids from your diet and environment are not effectively eliminated because of an unhealthy bowel, they become reabsorbed into your body, and eventually the calcium in your bones is used to neutralize these acids, causing bone loss as well.

Absorption of amino acids

The digestion of protein yields amino acids, and a healthy bowel helps your body absorb these needed nutrients. Amino acids are necessary for brain health and the formation of muscle, for example. Difficulty gaining healthy muscle weight is usually a result of poor amino acid absorption. Better muscle formation helps both the underweight and overweight person look better.

People with eating disorders often have very poor amino acid absorption, and forcing these people to eat more food usually results in excess bloating, discomfort, and water and fat gain—responses that, understandably, often result in the patient quitting the eating disorder program. The traditional advice for people with these disorders is wrong and destined for failure. The programs fail, not the people following them. And they fail because they fail to correct the underlying digestive problems these people have.

Homocysteine is an amino acid that occurs during improper protein digestion. As mentioned earlier, higher levels of homocysteine have been linked with increased cardiovascular disease.

Amino acids have long been used as therapeutic agents to treat numerous symptoms. While this can prove helpful, they are simply crutches that one would need to consume daily to maintain any long-lasting benefit. A healthy bowel that digests the protein that you eat, and easily and efficiently converts it into amino acids, is significantly more effective.

Manufacture of digestive enzymes

Some health books claim that if you do not eat only raw foods, which are full of digestive enzymes, you will die prematurely. I read this many years ago when I was very ill and it never made sense to me. Look at the Chinese. Practically all of their food is cooked, and they live a long time, longer than us.

When your bowel bacteria are healthy, you have a healthy supply of enzymes, and only *consuming enzyme-rich foods, like raw foods, is not necessary to sustain a healthy and long life.* Healing your bowel bacterial levels, which naturally improves your enzyme levels, is far superior to addressing this problem by only eating a raw foods diet. For one, it is very difficult to live in this country and eat this way. This can create a lot of stress and social isolation—neither of which are good for your health. Two, raw food consumption can help with enzyme levels, but it does nothing to improve the health of your bowel bacteria, which is the cause of your digestive problems, your unhealthy bowel. Digestive enzymes are crutches that treat symptoms and do not heal the underlying cause of the problem. If you eat only raw foods but do not heal your bowel, you run the risk of developing new, and possibly worse, symptoms in the future, due to your unhealthy bowel. Raw foods can also contain high levels of dangerous bacteria like salmonella.

Improved immunity (fights off dangerous bacteria, such as E-coli, staph, pneumonia, Lyme, and H-pylori)

It is said that your intestinal lining houses 70% of the immune system for your whole body. More specifically, a healthy intestinal bacterial environment is needed to fight off dangerous bacteria and other organisms. It takes a lot of good bacteria to fight off the bad bacteria.

Bacterial infections cause numerous symptoms and deaths every year. Every year many people die of pneumonia. H-pylori is a bacteria that has been linked to indigestion, ulcers, stomach cancer, high cholesterol, heart attack, and atrophic gastritis, is found in the stomachs of three out of five people tested. More than 25,000 cases of food poisoning are due to infection with E. coli alone, and over 90% of the bacteria causing urinary tract infections are E.coli.

Have you heard of MSRA? It is a deadly, drug-resistant strain of staph that killed three children in October 2007 and is said to kill 19,000 people annually. The Centers for Disease Control estimate that it could overtake AIDS as a killer in the U.S. This is just one example of the dangers of relying on antibiotics to protect you and not a healthy bowel; some deadly germs are becoming resilient to them. It is much safer to rely on your healthy bowel to destroy germs. Your bowel bacteria won't become resilient!

Food borne outbreaks—spinach, dog food, lettuce, carrots, etc. have increased in recent years. Currently we are witnessing a major recall of peanut-containing foods that may be contaminated with salmonella. In April 2007, the news reported that as we have imported more and more food from other countries the risk of contamination has grown significantly. They reported a $10 billion increase in imports versus the year prior, and also stated that in the last four years, there has been a 25% reduction in FDA agents inspecting our food. The annual number of deaths from food borne illnesses in the United States alone is over 5,000.

Vitamin D stimulates the production of the antimicrobial cathe-licidin, which targets bacteria, viruses, and fungi. Harvard researchers have reported that higher levels of vitamin D may reduce the risk of developing multiple sclerosis by as much as 62%. This may explain why people who have limited exposure to sunlight have been found to have higher incidences of multiple sclerosis. A healthy bowel produces these beneficial antimicrobials.

A client came in a few weeks ago telling a horrible story of a friend of his who was in a coma, fighting for his life after a prostate biopsy led to an untreated E-coli infection. I do not know the details of this situation, but if you are having a biopsy on your prostrate it is likely because it is suspected to be cancerous. Prostate cancer is primarily caused by excess testosterone re-absorption, a situation that only occurs when your bowel bacteria are weak. Likewise, an E-coli infection would only be deadly in a person with unhealthy bowel bacteria. The two are related, in other words, and this story shows the importance of treating the cause of your symptoms.

Not everyone who eats contaminated food gets sick. And not everyone who is exposed to harmful bacteria gets sick either. On trips to Mexico and other foreign countries with a higher exposure of organisms our bodies are not used to, not everyone gets diarrhea. I have been to Mexico six times and not once have I had an intestinal problem arise from my visits there. A healthy bowel protects you from these troubles; likewise, if you experience them, you have been given a warning from your bowel that it needs help.

In this country we are lucky that we are not exposed to more dangerous bacteria, like tuberculosis, or even parasites, like malaria, as many poorer countries are. But many predict that one day a strain of deadly bacteria will make its way to our country with devastating effects and millions will be killed. Your chance of surviving is significantly higher if you have a healthy bowel bacterial environment.

Will it be the Plague that killed scores of people back in medieval times? On January 14, 2008, an article appeared warning that the Plague, which is *caused by a bacterium,* is re-surfacing. On May 29, 2008 I read another article warning about a dangerous intestinal superbug, called Clostridium difficle or C-diff, which is resistant to some antibiotics and responsible for 300,000 hospitalizations in 2005, more than double the number in 2000. Scientists estimate that 5,500 of these cases were fatal.

Whatever "it" is, I feel very safe knowing that my bowel, and that of my children, is healthy.

The breakdown of gluten and lactose and the elimination of food allergies

Thirty to fifty million Americans produce insufficient amounts of lactase to digest the lactose, or sugar, in milk products. Between 1997 and 2002, there was a 100% increase in the incidence of peanut allergies in children. Gluten allergies are soaring. Twenty years ago when I was diagnosed with one I was considered odd. Nowadays, it's a common discussion. A client came in the other day and said that at her son's soccer game it is all that the mothers talk about. The number of gluten-free products has increased dramatically in the last few years.

Studies have found that mice with poor bowel bacteria were more susceptible to allergies than healthier mice. A study of 29 Estonian and 33 Swedish two year old children found that 36 were non allergenic and 27 had a confirmed diagnosis of allergy, with at least one skin prick test positive to egg or cow's milk. The allergic children were less often colonized with lactobacilli, as compared with the non allergic children in both countries. Allergic children had higher counts of aerobic microorganisms, specifically coliforms and *Staphylococcus aureus,* but lower proportions of anaerobic microorganisms like *Bacteriodes.* ("The Intestinal Microflora in Allergic Estonian and Swedish 2-Year-Old Children," Bjorksten B, et al, <u>Clin Exp Allergy</u>, 1999; 29:342-346.

From ABC News online, 2/24/04: "Treatment may reduce child allergy development." "Researcher's believe "good bacteria" may be the key to preventing children developing allergies. In the first of its kind in Australia, a trial has begun at Perth's Princess Margaret Hospital that involves administering dietary supplements known as probiotics, to babies twice a day for their first six months. An estimated 40 percent of children have some kind of allergy."

When someone is diagnosed with gluten, lactose, or other allergies or intolerances, most practitioners advise them to avoid these foods, eat a high protein diet, and take acidophilus, at a dose that, on average, would take two hundred years to heal their bowel!

If you have symptoms after eating dairy or gluten-containing products, these products are a trigger of your symptoms, not the cause. Many of my clients have been able to eat dairy and wheat again without any symptoms after following this healing program. When I was very ill, I went to the emergency room twice after consuming wheat. I now consume wheat daily with zero ill effects.

Food allergies can be deadly in the immediate term. In the long-term, if you avoid a food you are allergic or sensitive to and do not address the cause of the problem—especially if you incorporate a high protein diet, as most people do—you will end up with more serious problems down the road as a result of a continually worsening of your bowel and body health.

Manufacture of melatonin

There is 400 times more melatonin in your bowel than in your pineal gland, the gland most discussed in relation to melatonin production. While melatonin is most well known to help with *insomnia,* it also helps with the production of hydrochloric acid and pepsin, two important enzymes needed for the *proper digestion of protein.* It improves circulation and activity of the bowel. Traveling can affect these levels and low levels of melatonin are one reason why many suffer from jet lag and *"traveler's constipation."* Melatonin affects bicarbonate production, an alkaline agent that helps to buffer the harmful effects of excess acids. It acts as an antioxidant. It protects your bowel from *ulcer formation* and has been found to protect your pancreas as well. In large doses, it has been shown to shrink the regression of *cancer.* This may be one reason why people who work night shifts have higher cancer rates, as melatonin production naturally occurs in the evening when it becomes dark.

Manufacture of vitamin K and other nutrients

Vitamin K is needed for *healthy clotting of your blood,* so you don't bleed to death. Vitamin K is also used to help bind calcium to bone which helps build *strong bones.*

A healthy bowel affects other nutrient levels as well, including some of the other B-vitamins. Candida, yeast that multiplies in your bowel when the beneficial bacterial levels are low, produces an enzyme called thiaminase that destroys Vitamin B-1 in your bowel. When your bowel is healthy, you will have healthy levels of Vitamin B1. This vitamin is needed to neutralize the lactic acid produced during exercise, *preventing soreness and improving recovery.* It also affects *energy, growth, learning capacity, circulation, carbohydrate metabolism,* and is needed for *normal muscle tone of your intestines, stomach, and heart.*

Removal of cholesterol

A study in the Journal of Dairy Science, March 2000, showed a 17% improvement in the ration of HDL to LDL in mice that were fed a probiotic. Excess cholesterol, like any waste product, depends on a healthy bowel for its elimination; to prevent it from being reabsorbed into your blood and, ultimately, into your arteries, where it can kill you.

Healthy bacteria help your body break down bile, and bile also helps with the removal of excess cholesterol. High bilirubin levels in blood work and/or yellow in the whites of your eyes are symptoms of improper bile break down and therefore of an unhealthy bowel.

Finally, when your bowel bacterial environment is healthy, you eliminate the acids that cause your body to manufacture more cholesterol to buffer these acids in the first place.

Removal of toxic heavy metals like mercury

Ninety percent of mercury is excreted in bile complexed with glutathione and cysteine, although 70% of it is thought to (undergo enterohepatic cycling) and be returned to your liver. Mercury cannot get out of your body if your bowel is unhealthy. Glutathione and cysteine bind to mercury in your blood and reduce the uncomfortable symptoms associated with its presence there, but this *does not* mean that it is eliminated from your body. *It takes a healthy bowel to actually eliminate heavy metals from your body.*

Excess mercury re-absorption is said to be the primary risk of vaccinations containing mercury and neurological disorders, like Autism, that are being blamed for this. Mercury is a poison that can damage your nervous system, kidneys and other organs. A healthy bowel eliminates it so that damage is not done.

Urine should be light yellow

For many years magazines and other media have promoted the idea that if your urine is yellow it means you are dehydrated. This information has been most loudly voiced to athletes in various sports publications. The solution given is to drink a lot of water, until your urine became clear. Like so much other advice we have been given, this is wrong, and ingesting too much water can be dangerous.

It is true that urine that is dark yellow, or that has a strong odor, is not healthy and that drinking water is helpful in these cases. It should also be noted that if you are taking a supplement that has vitamin B-2 in it, it is perfectly normal for your urine to turn neon yellow. It is *not true* that urine should be clear. That is not healthy. *Healthy urine should be light yellow. This reflects not only proper hydration, but also the presence of sufficient beneficial bacteria in your digestive system.* The beneficial bacteria create this light yellow color. Many of my clients have commented that their once clear urine turned light yellow during this process.

Removal of impacted material

Good bacteria break down impacted material on your intestinal walls so that it can be eliminated. Colonics and some bowel cleansing programs promise to remove this, but they do not address the cause of it, and unless you concurrently heal your bowel, it will return. A healthy bowel keeps it gone for good.

I have helped many people heal their bowel, and yet it is rare for one of my clients to experience the removal of large strands of black, tarry mucus and waste that is depicted in some colon cleansing programs. I think these cases are rare, but they sell books and supplements. When you heal your bowel with this program, do not expect to see this, and understand that the lack of it does not in any way mean that this program is incomplete, inferior to other programs with these exaggerated claims, or that you need to do any of these other programs in addition to this one to create a healthy bowel. This alone will accomplish that for you. The other programs will not.

Candida (and yeast, worms, or parasites) can't survive in a healthy bowel

When I first re-located my practice to Boulder many years ago, I gave a number of local talks on a variety of subjects. The topic that received the most amount of attendance was Candida. For several years after, I saw a large number of clients who had been diagnosed with Candida--usually by a chiropractor, nutritionist or naturopath--and had tried numerous approaches to rid themselves of it. As the years went by, the Candida craze diminished, but it occasionally finds renewed popularity.

Candida is defined as the overgrowth of the Candida fungus in your intestinal tract. It often makes its home throughout your entire digestive system. Symptoms of Candida include every symptom imaginable, including but not limited to weight gain, headaches, fatigue, allergies, acne, bloating and gas, constipation and diarrhea, and difficulty sleeping.

The common alternative treatment for Candida is wrong. I have read most of the books on the subject and they all pretty much take the same approach: killing off the Candida with supplementation, and a dietary approach that includes high protein, low sugar food choices. One line of products aimed to help with Candida includes a probiotic formula with a mere 1.5 billion organisms per two tablets and a Candida "destroyer" with high levels of tannates, substances that bind to bad bacteria and fungus, rendering them ineffective. The tannates kill off Candida, but they do not change or improve the environment in your bowel that allowed it to grow there in the first place. People using these products will need to take them for decades to keep the Candida away, a situation that is highly profitable for the companies who sell them. The paltry amount of acidophilus in these products would take centuries to heal your bowel, the underlying cause of Candida.

A high protein diet temporarily reduces symptoms of Candida because it stops the movement of acids into your bowel, where they feed Candida *if your bowel is unhealthy.* Unfortunately, these diets can reduce your symptoms of Candida in the short-term, but because they lead to greater bowel ill health, they also lead to greater problems with Candida in the long-term.

These approaches don't work in the long-term because the *cause* of the Candida is never addressed. You can kill off all the flies around your full, dirty rotten-stinking trashcan, but until you fix your trashcan so that trash cannot leak out and rot in the first place, another family of flies will eventually find their way there. *You can try to kill off the Candida, but if the environment that created the overgrowth to begin with isn't changed—if your bowel is not healed--the Candida will reappear. I have seen it happen many times with clients who have followed these approaches.*

This approach is popular however, and continues to be prescribed because everyone likes a quick fix. There is often an initial immediate improvement in weight and/or symptoms, and when in the long run the weight or symptoms come back, most people wrongly think they are to blame.

Candida flying out of my mouth

Twenty years ago when I was incredibly ill, I too was diagnosed with Candida. At the time I didn't know anything about nutrition and the physiology of the human body, so I too thought it made sense to attack the Candida, and attack it I did. I tried every Candida-killing drug and supplement available. I know of nothing that is used today that did not exist back then. When I failed to respond I was told that I was the "hopeless case" and led to feel privileged that my nutritionist had some connections and could smuggle an illegal Candida drug in from France for me. This didn't work either. In fact, there was great concern about the function of my kidneys after I used it, one of the known dangers of the drug. Sure enough, I landed in the emergency room with kidney problems.

Anti-Candida diets

I was put on a strict anti-Candida diet of animal protein, veggies and yogurt. One popular author at the time advised that this diet not be followed longer than three weeks (I guess the red alert should have gone off then!), but I was encouraged to go longer because I was not responding. I was becoming more ill by the moment. Eventually I became so disabled that common sense took over, or at the very least, I decided to do the opposite of what I had been doing. This meant stopping all of the Candida supplements and following a diet of *no* animal protein. Mostly I ate vegetables and millet. I improved dramatically. I was not yet completely free of Candida and my bowel was still unhealthy, but I was definitely much better than I had been.

Many years later while studying to be a nutritionist, I was working for a chiropractor and was asked to go to a seminar for the chiropractic profession. The author of the Candida book that I had followed when I was very ill was there. At the time I was very angry and let him know how I felt. By this time I knew enough about health and nutrition to know that his advice was dangerous. This man was at least 60 pounds overweight, with a protruding "beer belly," or should I say "Candida belly." Not the person to be taking advice from on healing the digestive system, but he sold many books, and unfortunately many people, out of desperation, bought and followed his advice. The newer books that are written today on Candida are not as extreme as his was, and some use this as an argument of their superiority, but the approach is still wrong. It may be *less* dangerous, but it is still dangerous, and bound to fail in the long run.

In my office I rarely utter the word Candida because I don't want someone to focus on it, and I don't want to risk having him or her pick up a lousy Candida books. But the fact is, I would estimate that all of my clients have Candida overgrowth. Likewise, *this program will permanently eliminate 100% of the excess Candida from your body.*

By healing your bowel and re-establishing an ideal bacterial environment within it, you are fixing the holes in your trashcan, eliminating excess acidity in your bowel, and eliminating the "food" for the Candida. If all of the acids in your bowel are completely and efficiently eliminated, there are none left over to promote the growth of Candida. This can be a lengthy process compared to taking a Candida-killing drug, which "miraculously" kills off your Candida in two weeks. It is also an extremely complex process; yet *attaining bowel health is your solution to eliminating Candida completely, healthfully and permanently.*

These concepts do not apply to Candida alone. Yeast, fungus, parasites, and worms—none of these will live in a healthy bowel. Parasites are very common in the U.S., contrary to popular belief. They can be picked up from water, food, insects, pets, the soil, and other people, for example. Parasite-killing programs advertise that 85-95% of American adults have at least one form of parasite living in their bodies. They use herbs to kill off parasites, but these programs

do not heal your bowel, which allowed them to manifest in the first place. They fail for the same reasons that the Candida approaches do, too.

It is claimed that before Louis Pasteur, the father of our modern germ theory, died, he stated, *"The microbe is nothing, the terrain is everything."* My analogy has always been, "Flies will not be attracted to a clean trashcan, but only to one that is full of waste." When your bowel is unhealthy and not eliminating acids efficiently, an unhealthy environment is created that is conducive to the growth of Candida and other unwanted organisms.

How Your Bacterial Environment
Got Weak in the First Place

The pH environment in your bowel affects how well your intestinal bacteria grow and survive within. Dietary acids alter the pH of your bowel and are therefore damaging to this environment. A listing of highly acidic foods is given in Chapter 9.

Pesticides, antibiotics, meats that contain residues of antibiotics, chlorine, NSAIDS and many anti-inflammatory medications like steroids as well as over-the-counter pain killers, and synthetic estrogen, as found in birth control pills and hormone replacement therapy, have all been found to be damaging to your bowel bacteria, too. Stress, all environmental toxins, and many prescription and nonprescription drugs contribute to its destruction, as these are also acid producing. This total acid load disturbs the pH of your bowel, creating an environment that encourages the growth of unhealthy (bad) bacteria and reduces the ability of the healthy (good) bacteria to multiply and flourish. It also explains one of the reasons why a high-protein diet, which is highly acidic, contributes to a worsening of food allergies, weight problems, and other health problems in the long-term.

Studies of swimmers found greater immune problems than average, and in 1992, a study done in Norway found that chlorinated water was associated with a 20-40% increase in the incidence of colon and rectal cancer. (Int J Epidemiol 1192; 21:6-15). Is this due to the damage of chlorine on your intestinal bacteria? My guess is "yes." Products that remove the chlorine from your shower and tap water can therefore be helpful to the health of your bowel. Likewise, if you or your child is a frequent swimmer in highly chlorinated pools, you might want to make an extra effort to heal your bowels. My son was on the swim team for five years and I always secretly hoped that he would give up swimming, which he did, as I hated his swimming in the chlorinated pools.

A study conducted at the University of Michigan Medical School found that antibiotics "seem to prime the immune system to overreact to substances." After mice were given antibiotics it was found that they experienced more allergies than mice that were not given antibiotics. And a study published in the JAMAA, 2003; 291(7): 827-35, found that *the use of antibiotics was associated with increased risk of incident and fatal breast cancer.*

It starts from day one

While the above-mentioned variables are undeniably destructive to the bacterial environment of your bowel, *the variable that most affects it is the health of it when you were a baby.* **Starting out life with a healthy bowel bacterial environment dramatically reduces your future health and weight problems.**

Everyone is born with inherent genetic weaknesses. Just because you had ten toes and ten fingers when you were born does not mean that your internal health was as strong as it could be. There are many different houses in this country, and they all have a roof and a front door and windows, but there is a big difference in the strength (quality) of them. Some houses will withstand a hurricane better than others. Some of our bodies will withstand environmental, mental and dietary stress better than others, as well. We all know of the person who doesn't eat well but has few health problems. This person was lucky enough to inherit a very strong bowel.

When a baby is born there are no bacteria in his bowel. Healthy bacteria are transferred to the baby through the mother's breast milk. The health of a baby's bowel depends on breast milk, and the longer a baby is breast-fed, the better. One-year minimum is ideal. One study found that when foods and nutritive liquids, such as formula, are added to the breastfeeding infant's diet, risk of diarrhea increases to 4.17 to 13 times of that of exclusive breastfeeding. Only when the baby is not breastfed at all is the risk higher. Another study shows that giving any food other than breast milk increases the likelihood of death due to diarrhea. The inclusion of solid foods in the diet of a breast-feeding baby increases the risk of death from diarrhea by 2.6 times that of an exclusively breast-fed infant. If cow's milk is added, the risk increases to 8.7 times, and the addition of cow's milk without solids increases the risk 5.7 times. The highest risk of mortality from diarrhea occurs when the baby receives no breast milk at all; a risk ranging from 15 to 18 times that of exclusively breast-fed babies.

In addition to being breast-fed for one year, it is necessary that the mother have a healthy bowel to begin with. Breast-feeding alone is not enough; breast milk from a mom with healthy bacterial environment in her bowel is required to get the full benefit of it. The more money she has in her bank account, the more you will get when you are a baby. Your chances of having a healthy bowel to pass on to your children, as well as your ability to produce sufficient milk and not suffer from painful breast infections during breast-feeding, decrease when your baby is conceived through fertility methods, as a healthy bowel bacterial environment is a significant variable affecting one's fertility. If you have conceived a baby with the help of fertility drugs, your child will almost definitively need help building a healthy intestinal system after he is born. Luckily you can do this, but it will not happen automatically. Specific action must be taken for this to occur. Also, if you have a baby who is at least four months old who does not have frequent, firm stools, you should consider healing their bowel, too, or one day, sooner than is necessary, there is a high chance they will have serious problems as a result.

The health of your bowel from day one is by far the most significant contributor to your current health and weight problems, and it is not your fault, your mother's fault, or anyone else's, if it is unhealthy today. Everyone did the best with the knowledge they had.

Studies on Intestinal Bacteria

Every week I review current nutritional health studies that are published in scientific and medical journals. When I find one that discusses the relationship between the intestinal bacteria and health, I copy it for my files. Unfortunately, there are not many of these done. A few of these are discussed below and elsewhere in this and future books.

Likewise, all of these studies have focused on the use of probiotics; however, it is the effect of probiotics—a healthier bowel bacterial environment—and not the product itself that is responsible for the benefits seen. Because *Bowel Strength* helps create a healthy bowel just like probiotics do, I am certain similar results would be found if this product were used. *Bowel Strength* is a specific, unique product that contains many ingredients and is not widely available, whereas probiotics are. They are also a more generalized product, and as a result, it is unlikely that a study will look at the effects of *Bowel Strength* specifically.

The problems with these studies

In all of these studies, probiotics are tested as "natural drugs," but they are not. To be effective, these supplements need to be individually prescribed in large dosages over a long period of time. Studies are rarely performed in the long-term. And if someone concludes, from these studies, that probiotics would benefit them, they are likely to discontinue them, and lose the benefit of them, when they do not immediately provide a reduction in their symptoms (because they wrongly used probiotics as a crutch.)

Where is that country?

Most of the studies published on the benefits of the intestinal bacteria come from another country! I recently found six studies on probiotics, and four of them came from the following countries: Israel, Egypt, Italy, and Slovenia. Two came from the U.S., although one of these was conducted by a medical doctor with the first name of "Itzhak," which sounds foreign to me, and I am guessing this man is from another country, one where health answers proceed profit. It is just a guess. The pharmaceutical companies, who would make little money on the sale of probiotics or *Bowel Strength*, are not nearly as powerful in other countries. Ultimately, the main purpose of most studies is for profit.

Studies offered the following conclusions

-- Treatment with probiotics may reduce mortality in patients with acute burns covering 41-70% of their total body surface area.

-- Probiotics may have a beneficial effect on gut permeability and increase absorption of nutrients from it.

-- Probiotics may help reduce the spread of bacterial infection throughout your body and help stimulate immune responses in trauma patients.

-- The doctor with the first name of Itzhak was interested in the effects of smoking on the microbial flora balance in the nasal passages, as smokers experience a relatively larger amount of acute and chronic respiratory infections than non-smokers, and he felt he bacteria played a role in this.

-- In another study, children with cystic fibrosis were found to have a reduction in the exacerbation of their symptoms and improved body weight when given lactobacillus supplementation versus a control group that only received an oral rehydration solution.

("Effect of Lactobacillus GG (probiotic) supplementation on pulmonary exacerbations in patients with cystic fibrosis: A pilot study, "Bruzzese E, Guarino A, et al, Clin Nutr, March 2007 (Department of Pediatrics, University of Naples, Naples, Italy, alfguari@unina.it.)

I have never worked with a child with cystic fibrosis, but I am certain that if I did I would find an extremely unhealthy bowel. I believe this condition could be reversed if their bowel was healed. I know a child who has this condition and this boy has terrible bowel movements. They are frequent and loose, which is a sign of extreme bacterial weakness. Nothing is being done to change and support this condition.

A study done in Washington, D.C., with the help of a naturopathic physician, looked at food intolerances and irritable bowel syndrome. It found that food elimination was more beneficial than supplementation with probiotics in "treating the symptoms of this condition."

It takes time to heal your bowel and body with probiotics. These supplements do not immediately treat or eliminate symptoms, and as long as studies are done that look for immediate benefits from using them, you will continue to be wrongly and dangerously led to believe they are of limited or no value. This will continue until they are understood and respected for how they work, and used correctly.

Most of the studies on bowel bacterial health do not look at the big picture

While studies on the health of the bowel bacteria are infrequently done, when they are, they almost always focus solely on the benefit that a healthy bowel bacterial environment has on conditions that have to do with the bowel directly, like colon cancer or Irritable Bowel Syndrome, for example. This reflects the lack of understanding that a healthy bowel affects *every* organ in your body and the health of it. In order for other studies to be done that measure the effects of probiotics on a greater range of health conditions, addictions, disease, and weight problems, the medical profession would need to first acknowledge that a healthy bowel affects all of these. Can you imagine someone suggesting that probiotics be studied in connection with alcoholism, for example? I imagine many people think this study would be a waste of time and money, or perhaps it just never occurs to them in the first place? If these studies were done and the correlation between a healthy bowel and all health, weight, disease, and addiction problems were proven, everyone would all be jumping on the "heal the bowel" bandwagon. It would also mean that everyone would jump *off* of many other wagons that, for decades now, have made a lot of people a lot of money....

It is unlikely that these studies will ever be done, so I invite and encourage you to get on this wagon now. Don't get left behind. And remember, *a lack of scientific proof does not mean that none exists; it can mean that the proof simply has not been searched for. In the case of a healthy bowel and a healthy weight and body, this is entirely the case.*

If more studies are needed, they should be done

I read a comment from a doctor who is the staff gastroenterologist at Denver Health Hospital, saying that more studies are needed on probiotics' effectiveness before the medical profession will be willing to recommend these products. Is this just an excuse not to recommend them, or is the medical profession seriously interested in learning more about them so that they can better help their patients? If it is the later, all I can say is, "So when are you guys going to do these studies?" If they were really that interested, these studies would be getting done. I have seen no signs of that, so for now, I can only conclude that this is simply an excuse not to look deeper into the value of a supplement that could put a lot of drug companies and doctors out of business.

If it gets done, do it right

If an individual or company would like to conduct a study that looks for the connection between a healthy bacterial environment and healthy weight and the elimination of symptoms, addictions, and disease, it is imperative that the study is done correctly so that the results are not misconstrued and worse, you are harmfully and wrongly led to believe that this connection has no merit.

A well-designed study would be long-term, or a minimum of ten years. This would be long enough to significantly heal the bowel and body of participants and also long enough to show that this is not a short-term, treat the symptoms approach. Follow-ups every five to ten years would be particularly powerful, as this again would reflect the healing nature of this approach. People treating symptoms with crutches would be getting cancer, diabetes, and having heart attacks, while those who healed the bowel should encounter none of these conditions. That would make a statement. The study also would need to be individualized. Because studies like to control every variable, and because healing cannot be a one-size-fits-all approach, we need to question the validity of our current scientific method when it comes to health and medicine and supplementation. Finally, any study that is done with probiotics or similar substances like *Bowel Strength* needs to incorporate strong, aggressive dosages of these products. If patients are given a "one mile an hour dose," they may not reach their destination after ten years, and would therefore be wrongly counted as a failure.

If now, or in the future, you read a study on the bowel bacterial health that implies that this is irrelevant to maintaining your ideal weight or to keeping you symptom-free and healthy, find out the details of the study before you judge its results. Who funded it? Was it unbiased? How long did it last? And what was the strength of the probiotics that was used?

And if after reading this book, you still believe that studies are your guide to good health, a healthy weight, and a long life, then I have failed in my mission to educate you, or more likely, you aren't really ready to heal yourself. When you are ready, come back to this book and read it again. If this is you, I hope that you do

Chapter Four

Why Vitamin, Drug, Exercise, and Physical Modality Crutches Don't Work

The vast majority of programs for reducing your symptoms, addictions, illness, and weight problems are crutches, and fail as a result. Their recommendations fall under one of the following five categories:

1. Drug or surgery crutches to lose weight or feel better

2. Natural supplements like vitamin and herb crutches to lose weight or feel better

3. Physical exercise crutches to lose weight and/or feel better

4. Massage, chiropractic, acupuncture, and other physical modality crutches to feel better

5. High protein, low carbohydrate, low calorie, wheat-free, dairy-free, or any other food-allergy or restrictive diet crutch to lose weight or feel better

I recently went to the bookstore and pulled out eight of the bestselling books on health and weight loss, and 100% of them fell into one of the above categories. You may be overwhelmed by all of the choices out there. You may have been tricked into thinking that these books offer a new, miraculous solution to your health and weight struggles. If a book is written by a famous person, with a title listing a famous place like South Beach, or an exotic-sounding spa, that does not make its contents any different or better than what is listed above. No wonder so many people have said, "Forget it, I'll just take drugs, eat whatever I want, and/or get gastric bypass surgery."

These approaches do little if nothing to heal your bowel or eliminate the acids that cause your health and weight problems. The program that depends on crutches will always eventually fail you.

Donna Pessin

In Chapter 10 I discuss the right and wrong way to use these crutches. I give suggestions for using them so that you can lose weight and feel better while you are healing your bowel and body. When used correctly, as a temporary crutch to hold you up while you heal your bowel and body, they are invaluable. This is not the present way they are being used, however.

The Dangers and Problems with Using Crutches

It is important to understand the limits of crutches so that you keep your focus where it needs to be—healing your bowel and body. Thinking that a crutch has healed your bowel and body, when it hasn't, because it can't, is dangerous. It is also extremely widespread.

The mop does not fix the holes in your roof

If you have holes in the roof of your house, the rooms of your house will get wet and messy when it rains. If someone gives you a mop, you can use this to soak up the rain and prevent the mess and destruction. But what if it rains really hard? One mop may not be enough to soak up all the rain. The more holes in your roof, the more rain that gets in, the more inefficient the mop becomes. Mopping up the floor every day gets to be an annoying chore. Most people will blow it off and not do it every day. The floors will get wetter, decay, attract bugs, and eventually fall apart. The carpeted bedrooms won't be helped by your mop, which can only soak up the rain on the hardwood or tiled floors. Therefore, the mop is helpful, but not completely so. It does nothing to fix the holes in your roof that is causing your house to get wet in the first place.

Crutches are mops; this program repairs the holes in your roof.

A dangerously false sense of security

A serious problem with crutches occurs when you do not realize they are simply treating your symptoms and not addressing the cause of your problems; when you wrongly and harmfully think you are healthier than you really are because your symptom or weight has improved while using them. This false sense of security keeps you unprotected from harm. If your roof has holes in it and you put a tarp over it (which does not fix the holes), it will get less wet when it rains, however the holes in your roof leave your house very vulnerable to falling apart in the future. If you think that your house is safe because of the tarp, you will face serious problems down the road.

Feeling good and/or looking good because you take a lot of supplements or follow a strict diet does not mean that you are healthy. For example, having your blood pressure go down because you are taking a blood pressure-lowering drug does not mean that you are healthier, and it does not mean that you will avoid early death from disease. Fortunately, or unfortunately, the dangers of these programs do not manifest themselves immediately. This allows many of you to believe that what you are doing is not only safe, but also beneficial.

This false sense of health also often leads a person to avoid healing their bodies. Precious time is wasted on the wrong road.

But I felt great/looked great before my cancer diagnosis

I have heard this statement many times. I heard it again recently from an attractive, fit, young woman who was recently diagnosed with breast cancer. It reflects one of the grave dangers of using crutches (she uses the high protein and frequent exercise crutches). *Excess acids in your blood trigger many more symptoms than excess acids that are stored in your cells. Yet, it is the acids in your cells that are the most dangerous. When someone has cancer or a heart attack, they tend to have a much higher percentage of acids in their cells than they do in their blood, hence the relative lack of symptoms.* Hence also the danger of assuming that you are healthy and your risk of disease is low based on your symptoms, *if you are using crutches to manipulate them.*

Using crutches does not "cure" you

Just as the crutches you use when your leg is broken do not heal your leg, programs that rely on crutches do not heal, or cure you, either. If you put a tarp over the roof of your house to prevent the rain from seeping through the holes and getting your house wet, your house may stay dry, *for a while,* but it has not been fixed. It will fall down sooner than one with a strong roof.

When you are cured, your symptoms, weight, addictions, or disease will never return. New ones will not emerge. Programs that rely on crutches cannot offer these results.

Mistaken belief that a crutch is healing

Many of you have been led to believe that some of the supplements you take are permanently healing your body. If it is not known that these are crutches, you could stop taking them and think they can't heal your body. If you forget, or stop, a supplement over the weekend, you can feel worse. Because you were misled to believe that the supplement was healing, you might interpret this increase in symptoms as a sign that the supplement isn't working.

This to be particularly unfortunate if you then come to the conclusion that natural health cannot help you with your ailments. It's kind of like the commercials you hear where people say they tried exercise and diet but still had high cholesterol, so that means the only solution is to take a drug. The exercise and diet were crutches that did not work; it does not mean that they could not heal their body and reduce their cholesterol naturally, and it does not mean that drugs are the only answer.

Easily led to try another company's product with "special" ingredients

When you think that a crutch is healing and experience a return of your symptoms when you stop or forget it, you can easily be led to believe that there is a problem with the quality of the crutch. This misunderstanding is a major reason why people are easily sold by a company marketing their crutch with the "this will work when the others didn't" approach. A crutch is a crutch. *It is not the quality of the crutch that causes your health or weight symptoms to return; it is because you were not aware of the limitations of the approach you used. If you take something that helps you "only as long as you use it or follow it (a diet)," the* <u>approach</u> *has failed you, not the specific crutch itself.*

Temporary healing

A number of supplements, exercise, and physical modalities improve oxygenation to the tissues of your body and stimulate healing, but this healing is dependent on the continued use of a supplement, exercise, or modality; your body's natural ability to sustain this has not changed, and the problem will return if it is not. Results are temporary.

Trading one crutch for another is not success!

If you trade one crutch for another, you have not become healthier, or cured or healed yourself, either. Giving up alcohol, only to become addicted to an anti-depressant, nicotine, or sugar, for example, should not be called a success. Trading your cocaine crutch for a high protein diet crutch is not success, and *won't* be a "success" in the long-term. This program will help you get off *all* of these crutches. That is success.

Using them gets old

Millions of you lose weight but fail to keep it off because the diet or exercise crutch you are using becomes difficult to maintain day after day. This is a very normal, human condition and it is not your fault when your diet, exercise program, or supplement program fails. The program failed, not you!

I recognize that the vast majority of my clients will stick to the crutches I recommend for only a short period of time. I try to help them heal their bowel and body as fast as possible so that when they do inevitably stop their crutches, they have a healthier, stronger body, and can maintain their weight and elimination of symptoms without them. *Most people won't take something daily. When you heal your bowel, it is not necessary to take supplements every day.*

You may miss an important one

One danger of relying on crutches and not healing your bowel is that you may miss an important one. I had a young client who had taken thousands of dollars worth of crutches over many years from her naturopath, only to be diagnosed with breast cancer. Turns out, the crutch that would have possibly minimized or eliminated this risk, wasn't one that she was taking. She had many holes in her roof and spent a lot of time and money covering these with tarps. There wasn't a tarp placed over the holes leading into her bathroom, however, so the bathroom fell apart.

Crutches are specific and only eliminate one or a few symptoms. Healing your bowel, on the other hand, improves the health of your entire body, and it eliminates *all* of your symptoms.

Forgetting a crutch can be deadly

Crutches are dangerous because sometimes your life depends on them, yet it is easy to forget or miss using them at times. If on the day you forget to put the tarp over your roof there are torrential rains, your house could suffer serious damage. The day someone forgets their medications for depression could be the day they take their life. The day someone forgets his or her blood thinner could be deadly, as well.

Stronger crutches are needed as time goes by

Crutches fail because while taking them your bowel can become less healthy, requiring a stronger crutch. At some point, this becomes impossible to adhere to. For example, you may find that you must eliminate all carbohydrates, or ingest of a huge quantity of supplements on a daily basis, to lose weight and feel better. As you reach a state of mass-supplementation or mass-restrictions, the chance of your sticking with this approach, and feeling safe doing so, goes down considerably.

Does a crutch that doesn't work hurt you?

If the crutch is not working, then maybe it is not helping either. If you take a nutrient your body does not need, does this put unnecessary stress on your organs to eliminate it? -- Maybe. If studies were done that measured the effects of long-term massive supplementation what would they find? I don't know. If you heal your bowel, you won't need to know the answer to this, as you won't need to take massive amounts of supplements long-term.

Time and money spent on treating a symptom and not the cause

When you use crutches and treat your symptoms or weight with them, the time, energy, and money spent on these often gets diverted from the time, money and energy needed for what is important, which is healing your bowel and body. It is in part for this reason that I try to find the best crutch for a client and help them eliminate those that are not working. This consideration also weighs heavily in the crutches that I recommend most to clients, as discussed in Chapter 10.

The Medical Profession and Alternative Health Profession are Both Wrong

There can be great anger, criticism, and defensiveness between members of the medical and alternative health professions. Ironically, while they are at odds with each other, they both rely on crutches to treat your symptoms, weight, addictions, and illnesses. Maybe the medical profession is upset because alternative people often act like they have better "drugs," or that theirs heal. I understand their objection to the wrong claims made of healing, and I can also understand their objection to the promise of "better drugs." Drugs are more harmful to your body than vitamins, but they are also stronger. I believe that most doctors simply want their patients to feel as good as possible, and many people simply aren't going to feel as good taking vitamins as they are taking drugs. The majority of you choose one or the other.

To reduce the criticism of each profession and more importantly, get back to taking advantage of and getting value from what each has to offer, they both need to own up to the limitations of their approach and stop leading you to believe that they are curing you, and that you are safe and secure under their care.

Using crutches causes controversy

Our current obsession with the quick fix crutch approach leads to a great deal of controversy and argument, and for good reason. Unfortunately, you all suffer from it. The bickering between the medical and alternative people is not helping you protect yourself.

When a mother claims that vaccinations caused their child's autism, for example, a controversy will, and has, ensued, for good reason. It is the medical profession that becomes most upset by these statements, and I don't blame them.

When something is called the cause of a problem, that problem has to occur consistently every time the causative agent is applied. For example, freezing temperatures cause water to turn into ice. This cause and effect relationship will hold true 100% of the time it occurs.

So when vaccinations are called the cause of autism, many medical professionals are disturbed by this accusation, because 100% of the children who are vaccinated do not develop autism.

The mercury in vaccinations, the ingredient that is thought to cause autism, is a very possible *trigger* for autism. A trigger is a far cry from an agent that causes something. The fact that vaccinations do not cause autism in all children causes many medical professionals to cry out that this is a false theory with no value. The fact that many parents have witnessed a significant change in their child's behavior after vaccinations that contain mercury, and that mercury is a toxic metal that has been shown to alter brain chemistry, means that the mercury is a likely trigger for autism. My children, at age 10 and 13, have never been vaccinated. So I agree with the risk inherent in them and support all parents who question their impact on their child's cognitive function.

But the fact is *a trigger is only disruptive when the underlying system is weak*. Not all people who are subject to the flu come down with it, for the same reason that not all kids who get vaccinated with mercury-containing vaccinations get autism. It is not the flu or the vaccine that is the cause of the problem—it is merely a trigger. *If the underlying health of the body were strong, these triggers would be incapable of resulting in a disease or symptoms, as millions of people and children have witnessed.*

When dealt with correctly, this controversy and the many others like it can be solved. When seen from this perspective, it can be clarified and accurately understood. When it is understood you can benefit from it. When you understand that mercury and other toxic agents, like stress, are simply triggers to disease and that by healing your bowel and body you are reducing and eliminating the impact these triggers can have, then you are in a position of power and control.

How Do I Know If I'm Only Treating My Symptoms With a Crutch?

Dependence on a drug, supplement, modality, or diet

When you treat your symptoms, weight, illness, addictions, etc. with a crutch, the symptom, weight, illness, or addiction will come back shortly after discontinuing the diet, drug, supplement, or other program that you are using. If your weight is down only as long as you exercise or eat a lot of protein, or if your depression is better only as long as you take your antidepressants, you are treating your symptoms with a crutch and not addressing the cause of the problem.

When I was very ill I had neck pain twenty-four hours a day. This lasted about five years. It was worse than horrible. Frequent chiropractic adjustments helped ease the pain, but it always shortly came back. When I healed my bowel and body, my neck pain became progressively better and I didn't need adjustments. Now, even if I am stressed or not eating well, my neck pain remains gone. I do not need to follow a special diet or use treatments to keep it away. The cause of the pain was addressed and eliminated, and as a result, the pain is completely nonexistent.

If you have to avoid wheat, dairy, sugar, and/or any other food to feel good, you are only treating your symptoms with a crutch. The same is true if stress triggers symptoms, like high blood pressure. If your house was strong and no holes were in your roof, it would not get wet when it rained. When you reduce your stress, you have reduced the rain hitting your roof but nothing has been done to fix the holes in it that allow the rain to make your house wet in the first place.

Quick results of one month or less

Healing your bowel and body and making it stronger can takes months or years. If you start a diet, vitamins, or any other program for symptom-reduction and/or weight loss and you experience results from this within the first month, you have simply treated your symptoms with a crutch.

Because very few of you will have the patience to heal your body and wait for your symptoms and weight to improve as a result, I have included healthy recommendations for using crutches in Chapter 10. If you follow these and immediately lose weight and/or feel better, realize that you have not healed your body immediately; you have simply treated your symptoms as well. *If you understand this differentiation, and do not confuse symptom reduction with healing, you are on your way to achieving success and a dramatic improvement in your health, weight, and life, with this program.*

Your elimination has not improved

Some of you have been wrongly told that you are already on a healing program that gets acids, or toxins, out of your body. In most cases, this is simply not true. Just because you do something that makes you feel better does not mean that you have eliminated acids from your body.

There are only four ways to eliminate acids: through your breath, skin, urine, and stool. Therefore, the only methods that help your body eliminate acids are ones that include deep breathing for the elimination of them from your breath, sweating for the elimination of them from your skin, drinking water for the elimination of them in your urine, and healing your bowel for the elimination of them in your stools.

I recently read an alternative nutrition newsletter geared towards the sale of numerous products the author profits from. In one section he prints an article from a man who speaks of the value of eliminating acids, or toxins from the body. His suggestion for accomplishing this is the ingestion of two teaspoons of sea salt a day. I love this suggestion and make it myself as well, but sea salt water does not eliminate acids. It buffers them in your blood so you look and feel better, but that is not the same as eliminating them! It is like spraying perfume on the trash in your house and saying it smells better. It would be even better if the trash were removed from your house in the first place. The author goes on to say that your body will only eliminate toxins as long as you keep drinking this, which should be your sign that you are *treating symptoms with a crutch (the sea salt water).*

Donna Pessin

When you heal your bowel and stop this process, your healthier bowel keeps on eliminating better for you! Your healthy bowel will eliminate old toxins and keep future ones out. You will not need to rely on salt water or any other daily supplement or other "thing" to do this for you. If this author's advice really were helping you eliminate toxins, you wouldn't need to take it every day the rest of your life, as the author has done and apparently plans on doing. According to him, he has drunk this salt water "every day for the past 27 years."

When you heal your body there is "an end." Twenty-seven years is not exactly "an end!"

Healing ends; treating symptoms with crutches goes on indefinitely

If you have holes in your roof and never fix them, you will need to put a tarp over it every day for the rest of your life in order to protect your house from the elements. This could be called an addiction to the tarp. Most of you are addicted to some kind of tarp or another—a drug, medication, alcohol, coffee, vitamins, high protein diet, wheat or dairy-free diet, low calorie diet, and/or exercise. Most of you need to use or follow one or more of these daily in order to maintain your weight and reduce your physical and psychological symptoms.

On the other hand, when you heal your bowel and body, one day you will be completely free of these tarps. When you fix the holes in your roof, you won't have to deal with protecting your house from the elements every day.

A few years ago I had a client follow my program for about six months and after seeing improvements, she stopped and went to another alternative practitioner who claimed that he could finish "fixing her" almost immediately. She took the bait and I did not hear from her again until about three years later. When she called me I found out that—surprise, surprise, and shock of all shocks—the promise of an immediate fix did not happen. I say this with extreme sarcasm, of course. She also proceeded to state that her symptoms that had improved while I was helping her were still better, but that the ones that had not gone away yet were still there. She came to me, drove down the healing road, and jumped off quickly. At that point she neither went backwards nor forwards. She was exactly where she had been when we left off. Had she been patient and stayed with me, three years later, she would have been done healing her body and be symptom-free. Instead, here she was three years later and no better off. In an email to me she said that she did not want to do my program "indefinitely."

98

I don't blame her. I wouldn't want to do something indefinitely to look and feel better, either. Thank goodness for this program, because with it, you don't have to.

Healing takes time, but at least there is an end. It is not indefinite. Treating your symptoms with crutches may produce faster results initially, but it requires that you adhere to that program forever. This is an extremely difficult, and sometimes dangerous, thing to do. Treating symptoms with crutches is indefinite. This program is not.

Prescription Drug and Surgery Crutches

Drugs and surgery are crutches that treat symptoms. They do not heal your bowel or body.

Drugs are easy to take and they are strong. Compared to natural herbs and vitamins, treating your symptoms with drugs is much easier, and results can be much more noticeable, as well. Given this, along with the enormous financial power of the drug companies, drug crutches are still the most popular ones used in America.

Drugs are acidic and toxic to your body. Over the long-term they contribute to more health and weight problems.

While drugs are acidic, if used correctly, they can be an invaluable and necessary part of the healing process. Unfortunately, the vast majority of you who use them do not use them correctly. For more on this see Chapter 10. The goal is to get off of them eventually. However, until your body is healthier, some drugs can be beneficial, as they may give you the strength and patience to heal.

Surgery is very stressful to your body and can make it weaker in the long run, too. It is also dangerous, as many have died during or immediately following it.

When the plaque in your arteries is surgically removed, nothing has been done to address the reason they became clogged in the first place, and so the clogging eventually returns. When you have a headache and take a medication to stop the pain you have done nothing to address what caused the inflammation in the first place. The assumption is dangerously and wrongly made that just because a symptom has improved, the disease or illness has been treated.

Millions of you are treating your symptoms with drugs and surgery, feeling better immediately, and avoiding the cause of your health problems. Millions of you are becoming sicker, more overweight, suffering from more psychiatric and physical ailments, and getting diagnosed with cancer at younger and younger ages.

Long-term effects of drugs

Drugs are acidic and they make the cause of your problem, your unhealthy bowel and body, worse in the long run. It is another example of short-term gain, long-term pain.

For example, the popular cholesterol-lowering drug Lipitor can reduce your levels of CoQ10, an enzyme needed for a healthy heart. Healthy kidneys are needed for proper blood pressure regulation. Blood pressure-lowering drugs are acidic and over time these acids weaken your kidneys further, the organs that are supposed to help keep your blood pressure down in the first place. This makes you dependent on these drugs.

An article in the *Philadelphia Inquirer* titled "Hormone pills may only delay effects," (Wednesday, July 13, 2005) *provides research that backs up my statement that taking drugs to treat your symptoms makes you less healthy and more prone to those symptoms in the long run.* The article reviewed a study that suggested that hormone drugs used to treat menopausal symptoms "might postpone but not prevent menopausal symptoms." (Of course, the only way to prevent a symptom is to heal your body, and drugs are not healing.)

This study involved 16,600 women, aged 50 to 79, who were given either Prempro hormones or placebos for up to about eight years. Eight to ten months after the study was halted, about 8,405 of these women were surveyed. Overall, 21 percent of the Prempro users reported moderate to severe menopausal symptoms compared with about 5 percent of the women who had taken the placebos. *The women who used the drugs had worse symptoms in the future.* This study suggests that the drugs made the women who took them less healthy, as evidenced by the significant number of women who experienced problems once they stopped the drugs versus the women who had not used them. *The healthier a woman is, the less menopausal symptoms she will have.*

In 2004, a British study found that women who took common estrogen-progesterone pills for more than four years failed to conceive for an average of 9 months, twice as long as women who had relied on condoms. Hormone-releasing IUDs and progesterone-only pills didn't delay pregnancy at all. Researchers can't explain their findings but U.S. experts refuse to blame the Pill. Hormones are flushed out of your system in two months after your last dose, whether you've taken them one year or ten years, adding confusion to the results. This "it is flushed out of your body so it can't hurt you" argument has recently surfaced in the vaccination safety debate too. What all of these people are missing is the effect of hormones, or vaccinations, on the health of your body. *Excess estrogen is particularly harmful to your health, and this harm is long lasting. It remains even when you stop the pill, drug, or vaccine.* This weakened body certainly would have a harder time getting pregnant.

False security

Drugs give millions of you the false sense of security that because you feel better, or your blood tests look better, you are safe from premature death.

When you take a drug that immediately lowers your blood cholesterol level, you assume this has provided you with a long-term benefit of less heart disease and death from heart attack? **But, at least 40% of the people who have heart attacks have medically normal, safe blood cholesterol levels at the time of the attack!**

The false security of drugs is also promoted to you when a doctor or drug company tells you that as long as your blood tests do not show liver or kidney imbalances, these drugs are not hurting these organs, and are therefore not hurting you. A normal blood test does not mean that you are healthy and safe from premature death. If you still don't understand this, go back and re-read the section on blood tests in Chapter 2. *If you are taking drugs and your blood levels are fine, it does not mean that these drugs are not harmful to your health.*

Big money for them, big risk for you

Pharmaceutical sales are the biggest sector of the biggest economy--health care services-- on earth.

In 1997, rules by the FDA for pharmaceutical advertising were loosened, and as a result, we saw a 400% increase in dollars spent on direct-to-consumer drug advertising (up to $2 billion in 2000). Every drug that makes it to market costs $500 million on average to develop. *The ratio of net profit to revenue is higher for drug makers than for any other U.S. industry, and has been for the past twenty years.*

This all bodes well for the pharmaceutical companies, but not for the people who trust that their drugs have been proven to be safe. The average FDA review time for all new drug applications dropped from 23 months in 1993 to 12 months in 1998. At least 10 drugs have been pulled from the market since 1997 for safety reasons. A study published in the JAMA in 1998 concluded that adverse drug reactions were the sixth leading cause of death in the United States. The number of adverse-event reports received by the FDA (including side effects and interactions with other drugs) more than doubled between 1992 and 1999.

Your risk of being severely injured by prescription drugs is about 26 in 100 (and likely more, as only 1% of serious events involving drug reactions are reported to the FDA.) Compare this to a 9 in 100 risk of getting lung cancer from smoking or a 2 in 100 risk of being severely injured in an auto accident. Over a lifetime of drug taking, the average American has a 26% chance of being hospitalized from drug injury. Long-term use of just one class of over-the-counter drugs—anti-inflammatory drugs such as aspirin, ibuprofen, and Naprosyn—causes an estimated 70,000 hospitalizations every year. Every year, prescription drugs cause one million injuries so severe they require hospitalization, and another two million drug-related injuries occur during hospital care.

I don't know the statistics for "severe injury or death" from vitamin and herb usage. Is it 1 in 1,000,000, or 1 in 100,000,000? These outcomes are extremely rare, whatever the number, and extremely tiny compared to the risk of drug usage. Yet, in my experience, the chances are much higher that a client will be concerned about the vitamins and herbs I recommend, than about the drugs they are currently taking. I call that "master manipulation."

Whack-a-mole

Bill Maher described the false sense of progress in Iraq with this terminology. For example, as more security forces were brought into Baghdad to make it safer, it resulted in less security forces elsewhere, which made it less safe in those places. Somehow, however, we only focused on the fact that Baghdad was safer and either ignored, or were ignorant, that there was a shift of danger elsewhere, which is, overall, not progress or success at all.

Success with drugs and surgery is similar. A drug might reduce your risk of death from cancer but increase your risk of death from heart disease or another illness. If drugs "cure" your cancer but you die from pneumonia or a heart attack, this is called a medical success, but you are dead, and I wouldn't call that a success.

Many drugs simply stop your body's reaction to un-eliminated acids. If you take a diuretic, for example, this causes water loss, but that water was protecting you from un-eliminated acids. It served an important, homeostatic function. Since the drug does not eliminate the acids that caused the water retention, your body is now forced to find another way to offset them. Another organ or system is called upon, and weakened, to buffer these acids and protect you. *The symptoms created by this are often called "side-effects" of the drugs.*

Your doctor is trained to treat symptoms

Your doctor is not taught how to heal your bowel and body. He is taught how to diagnose illness and treat symptoms with drugs and surgery. Likewise, if you ask him for advice on your health and weight, it will always be geared towards treating your symptoms, too. This is what he is comfortable with. For example, this advice may include exercise, reducing stress, eating less, and/or taking vitamins.

You will also encounter this with medical doctors who bill themselves as alternative. Some people believe these doctors are superior to traditional medical doctors. I disagree. Every alternative medical doctor I have encountered is focused on treating symptoms, and most of them include recommendations for harmful, high protein diets. You might be better off taking drugs and eating a lower protein diet than being led to falsely believe that the herbs and supplements are superior and safer, because coupled with a high protein diet, I believe this approach is more dangerous. **I believe it is more dangerous to eat a high protein diet and use supplements than to eat a lower protein diet and take drugs.** *The best doctors I have found have a traditional practice and are emotionally healthy and supportive of your efforts to heal yourself.*

On Oprah, Dr. Oz said that coffee is good for you and that you should drink skim milk and red wine every day, too. He admitted that coffee is a drug (he is a medical doctor, after all), and that it can help reduce liver cancer and the symptoms of Alzheimer's and Parkinson's disease. He said that even though it has side effects, it is okay to drink coffee as long as you are not having any. These comments are a prime example of the dangers of listening to a doctor's advice on health and diet. Coffee is highly acidic and very bad for your health in the long run. As a stimulant, it can help minimize certain symptoms, just like any drug. But like all drugs, the short-term reduction in symptoms will be followed by a long-term health crisis, and greater health and weight problems due to the acidic damage of the drug, or coffee, on your body. He also recommends a baby aspirin every day. Baby aspirin is also acidic, and in the long-term it will make your health worse. A healthy bowel and the elimination of accumulated acidity will eliminate inflammation and heart disease. The baby aspirin treats the symptoms of inflammation without addressing the cause of it. This theme is everywhere in the medical profession, and it's something you need to be particularly careful about any time a medical doctor gives nutritional advice.

Do not expect your doctor to have the knowledge or experience to comment on the information in this book. Your doctor is likely more intelligent than I am, and I give him that. I cannot prescribe drugs or diagnose complicated illnesses and I give him that too. He is an expert at interpreting blood tests. I am not. He is also an expert on treating symptoms with drugs and surgery. I am an expert on healing your bowel and body.

Vitamin, Supplement, and Herb Crutches

Americans spent more than $10 billion on supplements in 1999 (Hartman Group) and $30 billion on alternative therapies. *Alternative health care is a multibillion-dollar a year industry, but we are not getting multibillion-dollar a year results.* Our weight continues to increase and our health continues to worsen.

Scientific studies show that people who ingest large amounts of supplements die at about the same age as people who take none. While people who take these may feel better, when you heal your bowel, you will feel better *and* live longer.

The majority of the vitamins, supplements, and herbs that you take are still only crutches that treat symptoms, just like drugs, but they are less damaging to your health and do not contribute to making the cause of your health and weigh problems worse.

Just because you feel better after taking a supplement does not mean that you are healthier. You are healthier if you feel just as good when you stop the supplement. You shouldn't need supplements. If you have fewer colds while taking them that is great, but it does not mean that you have healed your immune system. You have healed your immune system when these colds no longer occur and you are *not* taking supplements.

If the supplement does not cause an improved elimination of acids from your body then it is not permanently healing you. For example, if your liver is weak and depleted—a condition caused by un-eliminated acids—the herb Milk Thistle can give nourishment to it, but it will not address the cause of the weakness in the first place. It cannot heal your bowel so that acids are eliminated and no longer weakening your liver.

When you heal your body, you won't need vitamins, herbs, or any other supplements to look and feel great.

Alternative practitioners treat symptoms too, but with "drugs" that are natural

Naturopaths, acupuncturists, chiropractors, and like-minded professionals are trained to treat symptoms, too. They are not trained to heal your bowel and body. The difference between them and medical doctors is that the drugs they recommend to treat symptoms are natural and non-toxic, yet most of these professionals act as though they are doing much more for you. I disagree. When they act as though they are helping you heal your body, they are putting you in danger. *If they recommend high-protein diets, and many of them do, you may have been safer going to a conventional doctor instead.*

The Naturopathic Doctor News & Review is a prominent publication that aims to educate and market to members of the naturopathic and alternative health professions. It features articles and advertisements for programs and products to treat your symptoms. It shows pictures of Naturopathic doctors in medical lab coats, playing "doctor." And an article in the 2006 edition concerning cancer stated that, "Most alternative treatments are aimed at accomplishing the same goals as conventional treatment—killing cancer cells, or at least interfering in the cancer progression process—by using safer, natural substances and with fewer side effects."

As stated in another recent article from this journal: "You must supplement your diet if you wish to resist disease." This is the prevailing thought and practice of these professionals. They themselves follow it. In a recent article about a practitioner named Physician of the Year by the American Association of Naturopathic Physicians, when he was asked what supplements he takes he replied, "I take a pile every day, and the more toxic the patients I work with, the bigger that pile gets." In another article, a practitioner states that the usual recommendation for melatonin use is 3 milligrams/day, but that he has his cancer patients take 50 mg/day, and that he uses 9 mg every night. This is a pretty large amount. *It is 9mg a night more than my clients need when they heal their bowel.*

High-priced supplements, multi-level marketing companies, and additional profit centers

These monthly publications often advertise the benefit of selling supplements as an "additional profit center." Many alternative practitioners incorporate supplement sales in their practices because it can generate a significant increase in their revenue. The mark-up on supplements is high, and they can make a lot of money selling them.

I am certain that most practitioners are honest and well intentioned when they sell you supplements, but I have met many who are not. Be careful. Supplements should be sold solely if they benefit you; the goal should not be to make extra money from them. It is fine if that happens, but to have this as an advertised benefit stimulates dishonest behavior among some of the people who sell them. (Of course, this happens in the medical profession as well. A client, who came to me after a decade of alternative therapies failed to cure her of her immune disorder, overheard a disturbing conversation by an alternative doctor who she worked with many years ago. She was at a hotel in Manhattan and recognized this man, to whom she gave a lot of money, time, and trust. He was speaking to someone about a revolutionary stem cell therapy and the dominant idea expressed during this conversation was the opportunity to make a lot of money from this therapy. She was appalled that the main excitement over this therapy was money, and not the potential to help others....)

Many of the products alternative practitioners carry are no better than the ones you can get at health food stores, but at less cost to you. There are no magic supplements. If I sell someone on the advantage of using a crutch, say vitamin B-12, I always tell them that I have one but that it is no better than what they can find for themselves at the health food store. Some practitioners make you feel differently.

Sometimes you get a better quality supplement for the money, but not all of the supplements that cost more are worth the price. In some cases, the higher price is charged because of a person's insecurity about vitamins and the mistaken belief that just because their chiropractor sells it, it is better than an equivalent product at the health food store. In general, supplements that you purchase from alternative practitioners and multi-level marketing companies are over priced because they get away with it. In all of the years that I have done this work, I have found that the supplements that are sold at the health food store are just as effective as the ones that someone else will try to sell you.

Practitioners who depend on crutches get cancer and have heart attacks

The doctor you give your power to may die prematurely of cancer or heart disease. Thousands of them have. This happens to alternative practitioners too; practitioners who are following the advice that they are giving to you! I am reading the story of a Naturopath who was diagnosed with endometrial cancer three years ago. She has been practicing naturopathic medicine and dispensing advice for over twenty years. I would not want to take advice from someone like this. I have always told my clients, "If I ever get cancer or have a heart attack, stop listening to me!"

Why scientific studies lead to the improper use of supplements and minimal results

People keep buying into the idea that there is a magic supplement that will work in part because they've heard of wonderful results of their use in studies publicized on television and in magazines.

The results of many published studies that are promoted on television, in books, and magazines are vague and over-stated. I am looking at one that tested 193 people. Results in this study found that symptoms occurred in only 7% of these people when they took a certain vitamin versus 14% of those people who did not take the vitamin. In other words, there was a 7% improvement, which means that only 14 of the 193 people in the study showed "improvement," whatever that means, with the vitamin. That's not many, and yet a study like this will generate recommendations that people with that particular symptom take that particular vitamin "because it has been shown to be beneficial," and many will be sold.

Long ago, I made the commitment to find a natural program that helps 100% of the people following it, not 7%. As a result, this program is different than what you have heard, but what you have heard is based on studies, like that one above, which only benefit a minimal number of people.

Extremely large amounts of supplements are also used in many of these studies because the goal is to see a result as soon as possible. The sooner an improvement is seen, the less expensive the study is. But in reality, when a result is published, you are never told how much of a nutrient the participants took; you are just told that taking a nutrient will help a particular problem. When you enter the store to buy this nutrient, you buy whatever is available at the dosage the company feels is appropriate, even though this is often *much* lower than what the study used, and your response will also be much different (not as favorable). *Supplements only reduce your symptoms if the right amount is taken.*

The trend towards higher nutrient intakes

Over the years, the recommended dosage of supplements has steadily increased. For example, when I was ill, a standard recommended dosage of acidophilus was about 10 million organisms a day; today it is 3 billion a day. This is an enormous increase. And while I took massive supplementation when I was ill, it was considered extremely revolutionary and uncommon. Today it is much more widespread.

The reason we have seen a greater response and benefit from massive nutrient supplementation is because our bodies are becoming increasingly less healthy and more acidic. *The less healthy your bowel is, and the more acids you accumulate, the more nutrients you need to look and feel better.* The problem is, most of you who take supplements don't get that they are crutches and that they will need to take them long-term, and eventually at even higher doses, just like medications, to maintain a reduction in your symptoms. If you don't eliminate acids from your body, more will eventually accumulate, and you'll eventually need a higher dose to get the same relief.

You become addicted to them, which is fine and profitable for the supplement companies and others who sell them. I've seen this happen with many clients. At some point, the larger amounts needed to achieve the same results is very hard to maintain daily, and this person seeks a new answer to their problems— luckily for them, when it lands them in my office.

When I was very ill I took thousands of dollars worth of supplements yet saw no improvements in my symptoms or health. At one point I was sold on the miracles of mega-nutrient supplement through an I.V. Once again, I thought I had found the answer. I spent many hours in an office hooked up to an I.V. while mega-nutrients were dripped into my veins. I was ill and acidic enough that even this did not help. A few years ago, I saw that this protocol had made its way here to Boulder.

I believe that until we start addressing the cause of our health and weight problems this trend to higher nutrient intakes will continue, but to a limit. Who wants to need an I.V. every week to feel better? Worse, because you are only treating the symptoms of your problems, eventually even these won't help, as was my experience. Then you will find that all of that time and money was a waste. Also, many of my clients are concerned once supplement usage enters into the mega-zone.

Eliminate acids to reduce your nutrient needs

As you eliminate acids from your body, your entire nutrient needs plummet (calcium, B-vitamins, vitamin E, you name it). *As your healthier bowel eliminates more acids, you dramatically improve your ability to absorb and utilize the nutrients that you take in; meaning less is needed to nourish you. Your body also uses up nutrients in an attempt to protect it from un-eliminated acids.* For example, antioxidants squelch the free radicals caused by excess acidity. **A body that is not overly acidic is a nutrient-rich body.**

The average American woman is advised to consume 1200 mg of calcium of day through diet and supplements, and yet osteoporosis, the disease thought to be helped by this advice, is prevalent in this country. On the other hand, for centuries Asian women have only been consuming about 400 mg of calcium a day, through diet alone, and the rates of osteoporosis in their country is much lower than ours. *We take in much higher levels of calcium to achieve the same or worse results, because the overall composition of our diet is much more acidic than theirs. I suspect their bowels are much healthier than ours, too.*

When I first see a client, one of the most frequently asked questions is about supplement use. There is a concern that I am not recommending multivitamins and other popular-selling ones. They are suspicious that I don't. To appease them, I tell them they can take all of these things if they want to. After some explanation, most of them decide on their own not to. Interestingly, when these same clients reach the end of this program, they *never* ask me "Do I need to take vitamins?" Maybe you, too, will only really get this concept when you get there too; when you heal your bowel and body and find that you look and feel better, and feel safer, than you ever did when you were on a popular supplement usage regimen.

Successful marketing strategies that continue to be very profitable

Millions of you have been sold supplements based on a marketing strategy that has been around for at least twenty years. Like all successful marketing campaigns, it will continue to be used by companies who sell these products and practitioners who recommend them, until you understand the problems with it and stop falling for their hooks.

Not long ago, an old neighbor called me and wanted my opinion about a new natural supplement that she wanted to start selling to others. *Before she explained the company's sales pitch, I knew exactly what she was going to tell me.* If you keep falling for the same story, it is going to keep being sold to you.

Below are the most common lines used and an understanding of why *all* of the products that have been marketed as "the cure all" have failed to deliver on this promise—and will always fail to do so.

It's not about soil depletion

For the last fifteen-plus years I have heard numerous supplement and herb companies market the need for their products with the argument that our soil is depleted of nutrients and therefore you can't get enough from diet alone. As higher and stronger amounts of supplements are being recommended, this persuasive argument continues to be among the number one reasons for supplement usage.

Our soil is not as nutrient-rich as it used to be. It is not depleted, however. A depleted soil would not allow anything to grow from it. *The amount of supplements recommended by most of these companies, and by many health practitioners, are hundreds to thousands of times higher than what would be needed if one were only replacing the nutrients depleted from poor soil.* It doesn't add up. For example, the R.D.A. for vitamin C is 60 mg a day. If the soil yields 20% less vitamin C in our fruits and vegetables, this would necessitate and increase in 20% more vitamin C, or 12 mg more—not an increase of 2000% more or 500-2000 mg or more of vitamin C, as is often recommended. If soil depletion is truly one of the main reasons to take supplements, then a 20-30% increase in nutrients, not a 2000% increase, would be sufficient to cover these losses.

In a healthy body it is very easy to meet your entire nutrient needs, *poor soil and all*, by diet alone, because when your body is healthy, your nutrient needs are low. Also, the most nutritious foods are the ones that I am teaching you to eat, and they are the ones that you will desire as you become healthier. Whole grains, beans, nuts, seeds, yogurt, cheese, fruits and vegetables are full of nutrients and can provide you with all of your nutrient needs. **This diet, along with a healthy bowel and body, dramatically reduces nutrient deficiencies and provides long-term health far beyond what one achieves with an overly acidic body and unhealthy bowel, swallowing handfuls of vitamins and minerals and herbs everyday.** In the long-term, you will also save money; because the hundreds or thousands of dollars spent on supplements every year will no longer be necessary.

It's not about absorption

Another popular strategy used by supplement companies, especially multi-level marketing ones, is the selling of their products based on a sales pitch of "it's all about absorption." It goes something like this: "All of the other supplements you have taken didn't work because you couldn't absorb them, and we have discovered a new, unique way to make these supplements much easier to absorb, so our products will work for you."

I first heard this used twenty years ago, and true, back then, there were a lot of very poor quality supplements on the market and increased absorbability was a value. But for the last ten years, companies who make these products have caught up with the increased absorption technology, and yet more products than you can count have promised to be the next greatest magic pill for all of your problems "due to better absorbability."

The reason supplements fail to become the magic pill that cures everything, and makes these companies billions of dollars, as well as the people involved in multi-level marketing schemes who fantasize about getting rich quickly and easily, is because they are crutches that do not heal your body.

People continue to fall for this argument, however, and my experienced guess is that they do because they are so convinced that supplements can heal that when they don't, they look for an excuse for why this didn't happen. They don't get that *the problem isn't the supplement; the problem is that these supplements simply don't and cannot heal their body.* The problem is that they are barking up the wrong tree. These companies can and do continue with this approach because it is the best thing they have found to sell their products, and every few years, another large group of people come along who haven't seen the failure of these products and are newly looking for the answers to their health and weight problems. There is a new audience to re-sell this pitch to every few years, keeping these companies in business, usually under different names.

Yellow pee does not mean you are pissing out your vitamins

This sales pitch of greater absorbability is aided by the fact that some of you have been led to believe that if your urine turns yellow while taking vitamins it is because they are being peed out, and these vitamins are not being absorbed. This is utterly untrue. Vitamin B-2, or riboflavin, can turn urine yellow, often neon yellow, when it is consumed. This is a normal reaction and does not mean it, or any other vitamins, are being peed out of your body. If you are taking a handful of vitamins, look on the label and find the ones with vitamin B-2. It is always in a multivitamin and a B-complex. Stop these and keep taking everything else and your pee will not be neon yellow anymore. Or go to the health food store and buy all of the other B-vitamins separately and take these, without any vitamin B-2, and you will see that your urine is not neon yellow.

If you do not need the vitamins that you take, your kidneys will eliminate them (that is, if they are water-soluble, like the B-vitamins). I agree that some people pee out their vitamins, but this is not because of the quality of them; it is because they do not need them.

There are no magic supplements

Every year at least several companies promise to have found the magic cure and sell a lot of people on this idea. I have been in this field for twenty years and I can't even begin to count the entire magic supplement cures I have seen come and go.

When you meet someone who has taken a supplement and it "worked," say his or her headaches became less severe, but you have no reduction in your headache severity when you take it, you blame yourself instead of the approach. You think and want to believe that there is a different supplement that will do the trick.

If someone takes a supplement and gets results when you don't, consider that they are likely doing something else along with it to get improvements, and they have simply told you that it was the supplement that helped. I had a client who came to me after he was diagnosed with diabetes and high blood pressure. He had started medications for both of these conditions and had also started consuming kombucha tea, a black tea made with a mushroom starter that is touted as a magic cure-all. He was feeling much better and in his words, this was attributable to the tea. Medications are widely used because they make you feel better, but he didn't give these any credit. He wanted to believe he could heal his body easily and quickly and that this tea was doing this for him. (So he took this magical road and got off of my road.) The story he was telling was one of the magic mushroom tea, which is a misleading story, but one that many will buy. Kombucha tea is a healthy beverage and it is great to consume, but it cannot quickly and easily heal your bowel or body. (This client recently returned to me in worse health than ever...)

Many practitioners give their clients supplements *along with diet recommendations that often are low in sugar and high in protein.* These diets are like drugs and can help you feel better right away, so is it the supplements, or the diet changes that are helping? My experience is that without the diet changes, very few people will get the same results.

Another reason someone may get a result with a supplement when another person doesn't can be attributable to the fact that the more acidic and less healthy your body is, the higher the dose you will need to take to feel a difference. Maybe the other person was healthier than you, and therefore the same amount of supplement helped her. In other words, it was not a problem with the supplement, but with the quantity taken.

The miracle nutrient: coenzyme Q10

About six months ago a new client came to see me and spoke of his interest in the "newest" miracle supplement, Coenzyme Q10, or CoQ10. I told him that CoQ10 was not new, and I proceeded to show him a book on it that was published exactly twenty years ago. I took CoQ10 when I was seriously ill. Back then, it too was touted as the "miracle nutrient." I felt no miracles after taking large amounts for a long time. Many others did not either, but here it is again, twenty years later, because millions of you never took it back then and experienced failure with it. There is a new marketplace to sell millions of dollars more of it to all of you who think it is a new, miraculous discovery.

Is there any value to CoQ10? I believe so. Like all of the other crutches, *some* people will feel better taking it. It does not address the cause of your problems and if your body were healthy, you would have more than enough CoQ10 in your body without having to take additional amounts. Will the CoQ10 craze die off? Absolutely, and many other "miracle nutrients" will, one by one, take its place.

...Or exotic beverage

Is goji juice the "cure-all" that it claims to be, that for some reason will "work" when all of the other cure-alls have failed? I have seen dozens of "this is the one we've been looking for" magic concoctions over the years, usually from a multi-level marketing company and always short-lived in its fame. This one, goji juice, is one of the latest and greatest. It has a great name, doesn't it? And it comes from the Himalayas. And it is a simple quick-fix solution to your ill health. No wonder it sells!

An odd sounding herb from the remote corners of the world does not mean it is better than anything else that is out there and that it "will work." But it never fails. The more exotic the herb, the more we believe it is our magic pill. I link the kombucha mushroom craze into this category, too. There are many other ways to achieve the same benefit as this mushroom, but surely some believe in the mushroom more, simply because of it mysteriousness and oddity.

You end up confused

Sometimes we are inundated with too many choices. Often, this is simply a result of many companies competing for our dollars. Do we really need ten different corn cereals to choose from, and are they all really that different?

There is way too much redundancy in the supplement industry; it is one of the greatest offenders of too much choice. There is no benefit, or need, for twenty different brands of calcium on the shelves. I see clients who are taking five supplements that all do the same thing all the time. With greater competition come lower prices, but unfortunately, to many, this overabundance of supplements to choose from leaves them confused, and scares them from taking them at all. It also gives practitioners who prescribe them more validity than they deserve.

The fact is, most of the supplements that are sold today are good and will work *if you use them as crutches and take the correct amount.* When supplements do not work it is rarely because of the supplement used, rather it is because the supplement needed to be taken in a much larger quantity to help; the more broken your leg is, the stronger the crutch that is needed to get around.

Recreational Drug Crutches

Recreational drugs are also crutches. People use them to feel better. They use them to alter their brain chemistry. Like all crutches, one can easily become addicted to them and the reaction they create. Before I altered my brain chemistry naturally by healing my bowel and body, I was in love with recreational drugs.

Bill Maher cited a study that found that recreational drugs are less harmful to your body than alcohol and tobacco. Bill Maher is a notorious pothead, and I cannot confirm whether or not he was referring to only pot or to all recreational drugs, but to some extent I completely agree. Marijuana is less toxic than speed or LSD, for example, and it is less toxic than most prescription drugs. Because it is illegal, I cannot recommend it, but if it were legal (something I am for), it would be a great temporary crutch to use at times in place of an acidic drug. For example, I would encourage you to use it as a sedative to calm your fears and anxieties. It would replace other, more acidic and therefore harmful, crutches that you currently use to achieve the same effect. Marijuana is not illegal because of the harmful effects of it; the illegality is purely a political tactic.

More importantly, when your bowel and body are healed, all crutches, including recreational drugs, become undesirable and no longer needed to feel good. Your brain chemistry will be altered naturally and you will be "high on life." Now *here* is a way to win the war on drugs, and for much less money than our past and current tactics.

Exercise Crutches

Exercise is a crutch too. It can help you lose weight and feel better, but exercise does not heal your bowel or body. It does not address the cause of your weight problems. **When your bowel and body are healthy, you will not need to exercise to look and feel good.**

The primary benefits of exercise are an increased *metabolism* (the breaking down of fats into fatty acids), increased circulation, increased oxygenation, and an increase in pleasurable and hunger-reducing chemicals to your brain, like serotonin and endorphins.

If your bowel were healthy, it would eliminate the acids that cause low oxygen levels in your body. You wouldn't need exercise to stimulate increased oxygenation. If your bowel were healthy, you wouldn't need exercise to keep you thin. You would be thin without it. If your bowel were healthy, you would have plenty of endorphins manufactured, and your brain would be happy without exercise.

Done correctly, exercise is a safe, non-toxic crutch and has value for this reason. If your exercise program prevents or limits your likelihood of eating a high-protein diet or of using medications to combat depression, for example, it is definitely beneficial. On the other hand, nowadays too many people who exercise have been led down the high-protein path; seemingly many more people than those who do not exercise. Many personal trainers are under pressure to deliver quick weight-loss results to their clients. They have been taught how to do this; they are not taught how to create a healthy body. If you exercise among others at a health club you will inevitably be exposed to these diets and tempted to try them, more so than if these people do not surround you. **If you have taken up exercise and concurrently began a high-protein diet, you are doing more harm than good.**

Exercise is sometimes done obsessively to lose weight and keep it off. You can also get addicted to the effects of the serotonin and endorphins if these are not being produced normally and naturally, which only happens when your bowel is healthy. (Addiction is defined as: large amounts over a long period, unsuccessful efforts to cut down, time spent in obtaining the substance replaces social, occupational, or recreational activities, and continued use despite adverse consequences.)

I live in a town that is extremely athletic. Exercise is a top priority around here, yet I have numerous clients who exercise religiously who are very unhealthy. It is one thing to exercise because it feels good and you enjoy it; it is quite another to exercise because you have become addicted to it, or you have been fooled into thinking it will prevent premature death. Many people with cancer and other deadly illnesses have been dedicated to working out prior to their diagnosis. Because we have dangerously equated exercise with healing, doctors often say that these people did all they could to prevent their illness. Any disease or condition this person gets is blamed on bad luck or genetics. This is untrue.

I believe that the healthiest forms of exercise are yoga, Pilates, walking, and any other exercise that does not result in strenuous exertion and a hard time breathing, and does not make you feel sore, achy, or tired the following day. These are usually signs that you over-did it; that you created more lactic acid in the process than you could eliminate. An excess of this acid, like all acids, can be harmful, not beneficial, to your health and weight.

Massage, Chiropractic, Acupuncture and Other Physical Modality Crutches

I am a fan of alternative, non-acidic physical modalities for treating symptoms like Rolfing, massage, chiropractic adjustments, lymphatic massage, and acupuncture. I am not a fan of the fact that many of the professionals who engage in these promote them as healing and/or a cure-all. This is entirely misleading and minimizes their value. These modalities need to be viewed as safe ways to look and feel better while you are healing your bowel and body. It is dangerous to view them as the cure. They are very valuable when used as the crutches they are. *Like most herbs and supplements, using these crutches to treat your symptoms while you are healing your bowel and body is preferable to using drugs or eating a high protein diet.*

One reason these modalities help you feel better is that they increase your circulation, which provides some *temporary* help in healing. To maintain this effect you either need to rely on these methods forever—hence, they are crutches—or heal your bowel so that your body can eliminate the acids that reduce your circulation in the first place.

None of these modalities help you eliminate more acids. Eliminating acids heals your body. If your back feels better when you get adjusted but the pain comes back, only the symptom has been treated. Occasionally one of these methods, like massage or an adjustment, will stir up an excess of acidity. If this is not eliminated, you could feel worse, not better, after these treatments. If you feel worse, this does not mean the treatment is working or good for you. Respect it, and stop the treatment and focus on eliminating these acids from your body. Sometimes after one of these treatments, your stools become more frequent, albeit not very well-formed. Many of you wrongly conclude that this helped with the elimination of acidity. Frequent and poorly formed stools are signs of very poor, inefficient elimination of acids from your body.

Studies on acupuncture, massage, and chiropractic have found a reduction in symptoms with these methods. Keep in mind; a reduction in symptoms is not the same as permanently healing your body and eliminating the cause of them.

Ultimately, when your bowel is healthy and you are efficiently eliminating acids, subluxations, and blockages in your chi, aches and pains and sore muscles, and other symptoms that are addressed with these programs will not exist.

Shoving trash from the kitchen to the bedroom

With some of these methods, acids are simply moved from one area of your body to another. For example, with a massage, acids in your muscles are released into your blood. This makes your muscles feel better, but it can make other symptoms worse if these acids are not eliminated.

If your kitchen is a mess and you move this mess into the living room, your kitchen will look better. But is your house better overall? No. It is just as messy. The mess has simply moved to another area. The problem is, no one says hey, my living room is worse now because of what you just did. If you have physical work done on your body and your headaches go away, but your eczema flares up, for example, then this flare up is due to the action you took. If you prefer eczema over headaches, this result can be valuable, but do not wrongly conclude that the elimination of headaches is a result of healing your body.

If the mess in the kitchen was moved into the trashcan and taken away by the trash man as this program does, that would be productive, and your house as a whole would be better off from this action.

My Experiences

When I was ill I took a large quantity of supplements and spent a lot of money on them. I went to many different alternative practitioners and diligently followed their recommendations, but I never felt better. For a while I bought into the idea that I failed to see results because I was taking the wrong supplements. I now know better.

When I was ill I tried numerous physical modalities to get better too, including chiropractic, massage, and acupuncture. I had the most experience with chiropractic. Not only did I receive hundreds of adjustments, but I also worked for chiropractors while I was studying for my degree in nutrition. These very successful chiropractors always claimed to have the cure, and most of them sold some magic vitamin crutch along with the chiropractic care crutch. One of them is now pushing a dangerous, high protein diet. They are trained to treat symptoms, and a relief of yours is all that you should expect.

Eventually I stopped all of the supplements and other "cure-alls" and began healing my bowel and aggressively eliminating all of the acids from my body. I saw improvements that I never got when I was taking all of the supplements or doing the other work. My debilitating neck pain has been gone for many years, and I have not had a chiropractic adjustment for at least fifteen years. I do not take any bowel-healing supplements and I feel better than ever!

Vitamin supplements, herbs, and physical modalities are non-acidic crutches and can be *valuable if used temporarily as a crutch* while you heal your bowel and body. I encourage you to continue with these if you currently use them, or if you do not, to consider doing so.

Chapter Five

Why Diet Crutches Don't Work

Low calorie, high protein, low carbohydrate, gluten or dairy-free, food allergy, low fat, raw food, alkalinizing, and cleansing diets are crutches, too. They treat the symptoms of un-eliminated acids and the resultant weight and health problems. This is why they always fail you. You have not failed. **These diet programs have failed *you*.** Worst of all, many of these are dangerous in the long-term and contribute to more difficulty losing weight in the future, and a greater occurrence of future ill health and disease, as well.

High Protein/Reduced Carbohydrate Crutches

The majority of you are consuming much more protein than is needed or healthy. The majority of you use this crutch to lose weight and look better. Most of you are using a high protein crutch right now, whether you know it or not. For a definition of this diet see the section later on titled, "What Does A High Protein Diet Look Like?"

If you lose weight or feel better on a higher protein diet, it is because your bowel is unhealthy, not because this is a necessary or healthy way to eat. A lot of people also feel better taking drugs or drinking alcohol, but it does not mean these items are healthy for them, either.

The healthier you are, the less protein you will want or need to lose weight and feel great. This is one reason this program is urgently needed right now, because in the long run, these diets are very dangerous. They have been scientifically linked to higher rates of every disease imaginable and a shorter life. The early occurrence of disease in this country is horrifying right now, and bound to get worse, unless people heal their bowels.

Due to the overwhelming existence of, and misunderstands about, these diets, along with their long-term, dangerous consequences, I am devoting the majority of this chapter to these diet crutches.

Why do high protein diets help you look and feel better in the short-term?

Carbohydrates are converted into glucose when they are digested. Glucose is the fuel, or gasoline, that helps your body run. Your body needs energy from glucose and natural sugars to cleanse it of acids and toxins. It takes energy to move acids out of your organs/cells and into your blood. Moving acids out of your cells keeps them healthy and prevents disease. This process is uncomfortable, however, when the acids in your blood are not efficiently eliminated because your bowel is not healthy enough to do so. It also triggers weight gain, as your body retains water to buffer these acids and creates more fat cells to contain them.

Protein is *not* converted to glucose and therefore it stops or slows down this internal cleansing process. *It prevents the movement of acids into your blood. When there are fewer acids in your blood you look and feel better. This happens, however, at the expense of the health of your cells, and reduces your lifespan.*

If you have holes in your trashcan and you do not clean your house and throw trash into it, your front yard will look good, but the inside of your house will be a mess as a result.

The solution to your health and weight problems is not to discourage your body's life-saving cleansing process just because your bowel is weak; rather it is necessary that you strengthen your bowel so that it can get rid of these acids, as this program does. When your bowel is healthy, your cells *and* blood will be free of excess acids and the symptoms, disease, and weight consequences of un-eliminated ones. It is best to fix the holes in your trashcan so that your house *and* front yard can be clean.

If this has confused you, you only need to understand one concept: **you'll look and feel better consuming less protein** *only when your bowel is healthy.*

Glucose and fructose are not evil

If eating foods that are readily converted into glucose make you look and feel bad, it is because your bowel is unhealthy. It is not because glucose is bad for you.

Glucose is not evil. *It is a necessary nutrient for the preservation of life.* Your muscles, brain and organs depend on it for survival. When you are in the hospital and have an IV in your arm, it often contains dextrose, a simple sugar much like glucose, as well as sodium. I would love to see some high protein fanatic tell his doctor that he can't have dextrose in his IV. "Could you replace that with protein, please?" Even confused doctors who recommend high protein diets know better than to replace the dextrose with protein in the IV. Thousands of people across the country who are in the hospital would be dying right now if that switch were made. So stop thinking of glucose as the bad guy. It is necessary for your existence. It is the good guy.

When others advise a low-carbohydrate diet it is because they are treating the symptoms of an unhealthy and/or overweight body and not the cause, which is an unhealthy bowel. This is also why these diets fail to keep weight off in the long-term and fail to create health in the person following this advice. A healthy body will be thin; a thin body is often not healthy. To create health and ideal weight in the long-term, a high carbohydrate diet is necessary. There are thousands of good, unbiased, long-term studies that have been done on diet, and *all* of them point to longer life, less disease, and a healthy weight when carbohydrates are consumed as the main source of one's caloric intake. Look around at other countries who have consumed carbohydrates as their main source of fuel for hundreds, even thousands, of years, and you will find these people are thinner and healthier than we are.

Fructose, a sugar obtained from eating fruit, is also called "bad" because many people are intolerant to it. It can cause an upset stomach or even abdominal pain. Fructose is a healthy sugar, but like all sugars, it too is cleansing and moves acids into your blood to be eliminated. Cleansing foods only trigger discomforts when your bowel is unhealthy. *If you react badly to fruit it is not because fruit is bad for you; it is because your bowel is unhealthy.*

Eating carbohydrates that are readily converted to glucose does not make you overweight. An unhealthy body makes you overweight. A low-carbohydrate diet *will* cause you to lose weight, but not because it is healthier for you. Many drugs will cause you to lose weight too, but it is not because drugs are healthy for you, either. The longer you rely on this drug, this low-carbohydrate diet, the greater your likelihood of disease and death, and the harder it will eventually become to lose weight and keep it off in the future. The problem most overweight people face is that although they need to eat a higher carbohydrate diet, this is insufficient to heal their bowel, which needs to be healed in order to lose weight. In other words, a high-carbohydrate diet is never enough on its own to help someone lose weight. To lose weight and keep it off, to build health and reduce future disease, a high-carbohydrate diet needs to be combined with an aggressive healing program, as outlined in this book. When people simply try a high-carbohydrate diet to look and feel better, it seldom is strong enough to "work," leading millions to wrongly conclude that this means this type of eating is wrong. Don't make that crucial mistake. *You need to look at a high-carbohydrate diet as diet that you will eventually consume once your bowel is healthy enough to eat this way comfortably. You cannot look at it as a "diet" that will produce immediate weight loss.*

Refined carbohydrates aren't as horrible as you think, either

When you eat carbohydrates and they are converted to glucose, energy is created that moves acids from your cells into your blood. When you eat whole-grain, or unrefined, carbohydrates, they contain fiber, which helps move these acids from your blood into your bowel. While this does not necessarily mean that these acids will be eliminated once they get to your bowel, the fiber at least keeps them out of your blood for a longer period of time, and this results in less symptoms, blood sugar problems, cholesterol problems, etc.

Refined carbohydrates are low in fiber, which makes it harder for your body to move acids from your blood into your bowel. Overall, however, they are less acidic and easier to digest than meat products like chicken and beef, and are less damaging to the health of your body than those foods. (See Chapter 9 for an explanation of why low acid, easy to digest diets are healthy for you.)

Until your bowel is healthier, eating a lot of refined carbohydrates will make you look and feel worse. This will not happen when you have healed your bowel and body, and while they are not the healthiest foods around, you should be able to eat them without "reacting," with weight gain or symptom exacerbation.

We finally figured out we need good fats, and we'll eventually get it right with sugar, too

One reason the popular low fat diets of the past failed to make you thin *and* healthy is because a necessary nutrient, fatty acids, was too severely and dangerously limited. It took a while for the general public to become informed that not all fat was created equal. You learned that trans fats, or hydrogenated fats, are unhealthy, and that essential fatty acids from flax oil and olive oil are healthy. In other words, most of you learned what nutritionists had been saying for decades; that there are "good fats" and there are "bad fats." I trust that the same education will eventually evolve with sugars. There are also "good" sugars and "bad" sugars. Eventually, you will be forced to judge foods and choose them based on their effect on your health, not just on your weight and symptoms. When you do, glucose and other healthy sugars will be recognized as valuable.

A protein deficiency is not the cause of sugar sensitivity

High protein diets are used more now than ever before to treat the symptoms of blood sugar imbalances. Kids and adults being advised to eat protein all day and are led to believe that blood sugar problems are due to insufficient amounts of protein.

When the high protein promoters say that their diet reduces cholesterol and lowers blood sugar and cholesterol, it sounds like their diet improves your health. *But many people die early that have low blood sugar, and blood tests are a horrible way to measure longevity.* Heart disease, diabetes, and cancer result from organ weakness, and a high protein diet causes organ weakness. *Your blood work does not directly reflect the weakness in your organs.*

Un-eliminated acids cause blood sugar imbalances, or blood sugar levels that are too high or too low. An unhealthy bowel causes blood sugar imbalances. When acids move from your cells into your blood in response to eating carbohydrates, your blood sugar can go up or down in reaction to these acids that your unhealthy bowel is not eliminating. *Carbohydrate consumption is not the cause of these problems; an unhealthy bowel is.*

When my clients heal their bowel, they can eat a high carbohydrate diet and maintain normal, healthy blood sugar levels. If you can't, you need to see this as a warning that your bowel is unhealthy and if you do not heal it, you are heading for a disaster. If you need to eat protein for breakfast and feel horrible if you don't, this is a big red flag that you need to heal your bowel.

Respectable, unbiased, long-term studies have consistently shown that there are fewer deaths from *all* diseases, including diabetes, when people follow a low protein diet. Low carbohydrate promoters have dangerously led you to believe that lower blood sugar readings always correspond with a longer life. This is factually untrue.

Your doctor may advise you to eat more protein to treat your blood sugar problems, but that is because doctors treat symptoms of ill health and overweight. In the long run, you will be less healthy and worse off if you follow this advice.

High protein diets and cholesterol reduction

The promoters of the Atkins diet claim that their diet is good for your heart because followers often see their cholesterol levels go down. *The reason these levels go down is because a high protein diet stops the body from cleansing. The cholesterol that normally flows through your blood does not; it stays in your arteries instead, where it can kill you! Anyone who questions this should have a heat scan done before embarking on this diet, and one later after following the diet for 6-12 months. The high protein promoters never made this recommendation; had it, this dangerous fad would have ended long ago, and many lives would have been saved.*

Dr. Atkins, who died at a much younger age than I would like to, had at least one heart attack while he was living. When Katie Couric interviewed him and asked him how that could happen, he didn't answer the question. Millions of people are following the advice of a man who had a heart attack at a young age. **In the last fifteen years, not one of my clients has had a heart attack, much less die from one.**

My local newspaper commented that the high protein craze fell dramatically "after a consumer advocacy group released a medical examiner's report showing that Atkins was overweight and suffered from heart disease. *Over the past three decades, a dozen expert panels reviewing thousands of diet and health studies concluded that Americans should replace meat and dairy products in their diets with vegetables, fresh fruits, and whole grains. None reached the opposite conclusion (i.e., that people should adopt a high-protein diet). As consumers, we need to be constantly vigilant for entrepreneurs who exploit our obsession with physical appearance to promote their profit-driven agendas. The price we pay, beyond an inflated food bill, is life-long chronic afflictions and a curtailed life span. Let's hope this lesson does not come too late for victims of the Atkins diet."* Well said! I am relieved to see that the high protein craze is winding down some, but it continues to be followed by many, much to my concern and disbelief.

In fact, patients with high cholesterol levels have less coronary bypass surgery than those with low or normal levels! In many cases, the more cholesterol that is in your blood, the less there is in your arteries clogging them, putting you at risk of a heart attack or stroke.

Also, health practitioners have commonly found that cancer patients have low cholesterol levels. One may ask which came first, the low cholesterol or cancer. Is cholesterol needed to prevent cancer? I say no. *Low cholesterol levels can reflect an accumulation of acids in your arteries and cells,* and acids in your cells make them more prone to be cancerous.

Dr. Atkins and Dr. Phil, two people who have minimal, at best, knowledge about nutritional science, have advised the public to eat high protein diets, and you are listening. What are their credentials to make such a recommendation?

These are two people whose professions, doctoring and psychiatry, are based on treating symptoms. Naturally they would recommend a diet that also treats the *symptoms* of weight gain and not the *cause*.

High protein diets and other blood work

If you switch to a high protein, reduced carbohydrate diet and any of your blood test variables improve, it does not mean you are healthier or are going to live longer! I'll state it again. When blood tests improve on these diets it is because the acidity in your blood, that can alter these variables, has been trapped in your cells and prevented from moving into your blood. This is a very unhealthy, and eventually, very dangerous situation.

If you don't remember why it is dangerous for you to rely on your blood test to assess your health, please go back to Chapter 2 and review the information on blood tests.

There was a man on Oprah who was following a higher protein diet and Dr. Oz commented *how much healthier he was because his blood tests had improved. Oz then said it was discovered that he had severe blockage in his arteries.* This discovery was made *after* the improvement in his blood tests from this new diet. You are not "healthier" if you have severe blockage in your arteries! *You would be safer, and healthier, if you had a bad blood test and no blockage in your arteries!*

Did the high protein diet cause the blood work to improve, but the arteries to become blocked? Given what I know, I would say that it did, or at the very least, it definitely contributed to this, but the doctors and promoters of these diets act as thought the two aren't related!

So why do doctors still give so much credibility to blood tests, you may ask. If your bowel and body are healthy these tests will all come back good. When they become unhealthy, blood tests eventually worsen. In other words, historically, blood tests that showed imbalances like high cholesterol have been associated, rightfully, with a higher chance of heart disease or other disease. Doctors could somewhat safely conclude that a person with levels out of normal range was unhealthy and at a risk for disease.

It is not surprising then that doctors will conclude that an improved blood test implies greater health and less risk of disease. *But because of the growing popularity of high protein diets, this assumption can no longer be made.* We have not had enough time or data to support this, but I predict that in the near future this discovery will be made. *Doctors will find a population of people—*

larger than has ever existed before—who are dying prematurely of heart disease, cancer, and other diseases that have "healthy" blood test levels.

I saw another one yesterday—a women in her late 40's, very fit, attractive, eating a high protein diet—who has had perfect blood tests each year they have been done, but who was recently diagnosed with breast cancer.

High protein weight loss diets

High protein diets reduce the movement of acids from your cells into your blood. If these acids are not eliminated, because your bowel is unhealthy, they will trigger weight gain and fat production.

Numerous popular weight loss books advise a high protein diet. Most of you probably have no idea that high protein diets have been around a long time. They failed before to produce long- term, permanent weight loss and they will fail again.

Why then do people lose weight on these diets, only to gain it back later? Why are these books written? As a nation we are extremely overweight and there is a huge market and a lot of money to be made in the weight loss industry. People love a book offering a quick fix. Plus, the authors of these books present some convincing evidence. And let's be honest, a high protein diet is pretty easy to follow.

...And every other condition imaginable

High protein, reduced carbohydrate diets are also recommended for neurological disorders, depression, addictions, allergies, skin conditions, arthritis, intestinal problems, you name it. Many symptoms can be reduced on this diet due to the prevention of acids released into your blood, but this is a wrong and harmful approach to these conditions for the same reason it is wrong and harmful to use them to treat blood sugar, elevated cholesterol, or weight problems.

The author of "The Maker's Diet," a book that claims to heal your bowel, says that the "over-consumption of high-carbohydrate grain based foods…is a primary cause of intestinal disease and other diseases." This is extremely ironic. An unhealthy bowel and the inability to eliminate acids cause intestinal disease and other diseases. *If this program really healed your bowel as it promises to do, this author would not be coming to this dangerous conclusion.*

Practitioners love these programs because they make them look knowledgeable and powerful. Practitioners make more money when clients get quick results. These clients never come back years later and blame their diet recommendations for their cancer, so it is win/win for the practitioner.

Short-term weight and symptomatic reduction; long-term struggles and disease

A high protein diet is highly acidic. Excess acids weaken your bowel and body, causing further damage to those systems that need to be strong in order for you to feel good and keep your weight down forever. For some it takes many years before this highly acid diet shows up as disease; for others it is "the straw that breaks the camel's back" and quickly triggers heart disease, cancer, and other serious problems that have been linked to higher intakes of animal protein.

The National Institutes of Health, as well as the American Heart Association and the American Cancer Society, have concluded that excess animal protein leads to higher rates of heart disease, cancer, osteoporosis and kidney disease. These organizations evaluate scientific, unbiased, long-term research and have found a strong correlation between higher intakes of protein and a higher incidence of these diseases.

If you are ever tempted to eat a high protein diet, do some research first. If you want the truth about what is good for your health, stop watching the news. The only way you will get unbiased information is by doing your own research and/or scouring the books on health and nutrition at the bookstore and health food store. While a lot of these books are lousy, there are a few good ones on healing the body that will provide you with information that you aren't going to hear on the local news, or in your local newspaper. In fact, I recently heard from a writer at our local newspaper asking me for ideas on how to get in shape for the upcoming swimsuit season. I did not return this call as newspapers want to offer readers "quick fix, treat the symptoms" advice. This sells newspapers.

University medical libraries and the Internet are two excellent places to find nutrition studies. For a study to be relevant it must include at least 200 people and last a minimum of five years, but longer is even better. *You will not find a single relevant study that has found that the more protein you eat the longer you will live.*

On March 24, 2003, a study was published in *Nutrition Week*, a government publication. For over 22 years 2,000 people between the ages of 10 and 70 participated in the study. This is a rare, valid study that includes a large sample size and long-term data collection. *Those who ate no meat (vegetarians) had death rates that were one half to two thirds lower than those of the general population.* Wow, that should get our attention. Did you hear about this substantial study or read about it in your newspaper? Why not?

Dr. Colin Campbell and John Robbins are two authors who have studied the link between increased protein consumption and increased rates of disease. They both have current books that I recommend. You can also Google, "BlueZone." An old client is a friend with the man who has been studying the longest living cultures in the world. The one common link is that they all eat a grain-based, or low protein, diet.

High protein diets cause damage to your health, whether it is immediately noticeable or not

It takes many years of cellular destruction before the ill effects of eating a high protein diet manifests as cancer, heart disease, or some other fatal condition. Each day that you eat a high protein diet this damage occurs, but because you have trillions of cells, it takes a while before enough of them have been damaged enough to show up as disease.

It is a blessing and a curse that acidic, harmful substances like excess protein do not immediately kill us. It is a blessing, of course, because it allows all of us to be human and make mistakes. It is a curse because the lack of an immediate consequence of these diets harmfully leads many of you to believe that they are safe.

Of course this is true of all harmful, acidic substances. When I was younger I ate horribly and polluted my body with a large amount of alcohol and drugs. I did not immediately experience a consequence of this either. I thought, like many of you do, that I was getting away with it. When I become seriously ill, I realized I didn't get away with it after all. Sometimes the consequences of these lifestyles take a while to show up, but there are always harmful consequences. Our bodies are simply extremely resilient.

More excuses for eating animal proteins

Because most people have an unhealthy bowel—including doctors and alternative practitioners who make dietary and other recommendations—and feel and look better eating a high protein diet, they have come up with many convincing arguments to eat this way. Below are a few as well as a clarification as to why they just don't add up.

Craving meat does not mean it is healthy for you

I hear this excuse all the time. When your bowel and body are unhealthy, you will crave many unhealthy things, meat proteins included. If you crave sugar or alcohol it does not mean you "need" them any more that it means you "need" protein if you crave it. If you crave protein, it means your bowel is unhealthy, and you better fix it.

Anemia does not mean you need to eat more meat

Iron helps oxygenate your blood. When acids are not eliminated from your blood because your bowel is unhealthy, your body may "use up" more iron in an effort to oxygenate your blood, because excess acids in your blood attach to oxygen and reduce these levels. If you are a vegetarian and have low iron levels it is because many vegetarians have unhealthy bowels, just like meat-eaters, and you need to heal your bowel.

We are not cavemen, thank goodness!

Proponents of these diets love to say that primitive societies died early from a lack of crisis care, sanitation problems, and infection. They claim that the meat-based diet eaten long ago was healthy and normal and that people used to have robust health. If primitive man had a strong bowel, he would not have died early from infection! Many more primitive men likely died from starvation or death by accident.

People also act as though the fact that cavemen ate meat justifies that "this means we were meant to eat this way." If you buy that, then you also have to buy that we were also meant to live in caves, because that's how they lived. We have a lot more knowledge and technology than we had back then and our lives have advanced and improved. This applies to our knowledge about diet and accessibility to a healthier diet as well.

Do not eat right for your blood type

A popular diet book promotes an individualized diet based on your blood type. The implication is that we are special and have special needs, and a lot of people like this idea. The problem is, while this book makes it seem like you are getting your own special diet, it doesn't really work out that way. For the most part, the diets recommended in this book are high in protein and "work," but also hurt you, for the same reason that all high protein diets do. In fact, years ago a young man with Hepatitis C contacted me but never worked with me. Instead he went to the blood type diet author. He recently died of liver disease. I've never had a client die from liver disease.

While the blood type diets are not promoted as high protein, and some may argue that one blood type is advised to eat a more vegetarian diet, my experience is that they all end up being high in protein. This happens because the book does not emphasize the amount of each category of food to eat, and the low protein foods are ones that very few people will eat, like quinoa, for example.

When I was ill I went to a nutritionist who gave me a list of foods I could eat but did not emphasize the proportion of each I should eat, either. The list included chicken, meat, and other animal protein, vegetables, and whole grains like brown rice, amaranth, quinoa, millet, and rye. I followed this diet and ate only the acceptable foods listed, but because I liked meat products and was familiar with them, I ate a lot of them. I thought I was following the diet because I was sticking to the foods on it. I did not realize that the intention was not to eat meat in the large quantity that I ate it; that I should have eaten much less of it and many more vegetables and grains. I have seen the exact same thing happen to people following the blood type diet. Everyone I have ever seen who was following this diet has ended up eating a high protein diet, regardless of his or her blood type.

High protein diets and athletics

My experience is that athletes also like to think they are special and have special dietary needs as well. Athletes benefit from a healthy bowel and the complete elimination of acids, too. Working out, especially if it is intense, has the potential to generate more lactic acid than your body can eliminate, a situation that occurs more often the weaker one's bowel. Excess lactic acid leads to muscle fatigue, cramps, difficulty recovering, and "runner's trots," for example. All of these conditions hurt performance.

An article in a running magazine said that many athletes experience decreased appetite immediately after a prolonged workout and will wait to eat. The author advised athletes not to do this, as it will lead to decreased performance. The author advised the eating of a high protein meal after working out to enhance performance. This of course sends the lactic acid into your organs, which is harmful in the long run, but eliminates the conditions of fatigue, cramps, etc in the short- term.

There is definitely a macho image associated with increased animal protein consumption and I find that many athletes, especially men, like to believe that they need more protein. It is interpreted as being "more of a man." Ironically, many male athletes have low testosterone levels, and testosterone is the hormone that "makes you a man." Testosterone levels are healthiest when your bowel is healthy. In the long run, a high protein diet affects these levels negatively, making one "less of a man."

Just because a diet "works" does not mean it is "right"

This seems to be the most popular justification for following these diets, which is that they "work." I agree. They do work. They work at helping you lose weight, but they also work at helping you increase your risk of premature heart disease, cancer, and every other disease, and they work at helping you lose weight in the short-term but struggle with it more in the long-term.

Still, we seem to think that when we follow a diet and get desirable results, this is proof that the diet is good for us. When people lose weight on high protein diets they even conclude that prior to the diet they had a "protein deficiency." If you snorted cocaine all day long you would lose weight too. Does this mean that you should? Does it mean cocaine is good for you? Does it mean that you had a cocaine deficiency prior to using it?

Stop justifying your weight loss and reduction in symptoms on high protein diets as proof that they are good for you. There is only one conclusion that can be made from these reactions; that your bowel is unhealthy, and unless you change that, one day you will be faced with a health crisis you weren't ready for.

As you heal you bowel and body you will lose your desire for animal protein like chicken, fish, turkey, pork, and beef. You will also feel and look better when you <u>*don't*</u> *eat very much of it than when you do.*

Or whatever

I am sure I have missed some of the excuses used for increased protein consumption, but I really don't want to belabor the point. **There is no valid excuse for eating a high protein diet.**

Fear of protein deficiency

The average American consumes much more protein than is needed for daily activities, so why are so many of you afraid of not eating enough? How many messages have you heard that have led you to become so obsessed and concerned about this? Who benefits from this fear? I'll give you a hint. It isn't you.

Do you personally know anyone who has died of a protein deficiency? It's highly unlikely, so why the fear? Do you know of anyone who has died of cancer or heart disease? Of course you do. *Thousands of long-term studies show that the more protein you eat, the more likely you are to die of cancer and heart disease.* Why haven't you heard about these studies? In reality*, you should fear eating too much protein, not too little, yet I have never met anyone who feels this way. By the way, the thinnest and longest living people in the world eat a low-protein diet. Did you know that? Why not?*

Many clients have a deeply ingrained fear of eating too little protein. I think this fear is largely the product of experience. When the bowel is unhealthy and people eat less protein, they feel worse and gain weight. This has then been misinterpreted to mean that they "need" more protein and the "fear" is perhaps not so much one based on a fear of getting in too little protein, as it is a fear of looking and feeling bad.

As my clients heal their bowels and become healthier and thinner, their protein fears dissolve, even though they are eating much less than before. It may be a while before you reach this state, so this information is meant to support you along this path; to help you further understand why the eventual switch to a lower protein diet is necessary and desirable.

Protein deficiencies are very rare in this country

The truth is, our physiological need for protein is pretty small. Protein is used for the building of body tissues/organs, while carbohydrates are used to meet the daily energy requirements of your body. In a given day, we expand a great deal more energy than we repair tissues. It's kind of like your car: Every day that you drive your car it uses up gasoline (carbohydrates), and refilling your tank with gas is something that you probably do often. Compared to gasoline consumption, however, your car uses very little oil (protein) on a daily basis, and you need to refill your oil tank much less frequently than your gas tank.

Protein deficiencies exist primarily in these select cases: in foreign countries where food supply is minimal and total daily intake of calories is very low because of it; in severe alcoholics who consume a much larger amount of alcohol daily than they do food; in chronic dieters or anorexics who, for months on end, eat 1,000 calories per day or less. In all of these cases, total food consumption is low, and deficiencies of protein exist *alongside* deficiencies of everything else, like carbohydrates, fats, vitamins and minerals. As long as you are eating 1,500 calories per day or more of "food," versus alcohol, sugar, coffee, or any other "drug," you are most likely eating enough protein.

A couple of years ago, a woman I knew asked me for dietary recommendations when she found out she had medically incurable breast cancer. She already had breast cancer twice. Both times, she did chemotherapy, eventually had a double mastectomy, and made no attempts to change her diet or health. While it is impossible to reverse one's health problems when the body is so far gone with just some dietary changes alone, and she was not ready, emotionally, to work with me, I responded with the recommendation that she stop eating all animal protein. This could buy her some time. Her stressful response was "But where am I going to get my protein?" This is sad, amazing, and frustrating. *Every study I have ever read—thousands of them—shows a correlation between lower protein consumption and lower rates of cancer.* Her question reflects how strongly and deeply these protein fears have been imbedded in you.

This woman never worked with me and recently died at the young age of 54.

What does a high protein diet look like?

It is amazing how many of you do not realize that your diet is a high protein one. I think this occurs because the promoters of these diets are simply not marketing them as such. There are too many negative connotations associated with this, so they have cleverly designed their talk to avoid this topic. Some of these promoters compare their recommendations to the Atkins diet and use their lower intakes of protein to justify the healthfulness of theirs. For example, the Atkins diet can include up to 60% or more of your calories from protein. When another diet recommends only 40% of your calories from protein, they sometimes call this low in protein because they compare it to Atkins. This is wrong. It needs to be compared to your physiological need for protein. You only need about 10% of your calories to come from protein, and if you eat eggs, chicken, red meat, turkey, and or fish more than one time a day; you are most likely eating a high protein diet.

When you consume a diet that includes over 20% of your calories from protein, this needs to be correctly identified as a high protein diet.

Sources of protein

The following is a simple guideline of the relative amount of protein in foods. Very few of my clients have been taught this necessary information.

Foods that contain very high amounts of protein: chicken, fish, turkey, beef, lamb, and pork (animal protein)

Foods that contain moderately high levels of protein: soy, beans, eggs, nuts and seeds, milk, yogurt, cheese, protein powders made from whey and soy

Foods that contain low levels of protein: grains and carbohydrates, like pastas, rice, bread, and bagels

Foods that contain very little or no protein: vegetables, fruit, sugar, coffee, alcohol, and soda

High vegetable intake does not mean low protein intake

Eating a lot of vegetables does not guarantee that your diet is low in protein. With a high protein diet, the percentage of protein that you eat in relation to the total amount of calories that you eat is high. Vegetables are very low in calories. Therefore, eating a lot of them does not alter your total caloric intake much, and it does not affect your proportion of protein much either.

For example, if you eat a diet with very few vegetables but a total caloric intake of 1500 calories, of which 500 calories come from protein, then 30% of your diet is protein. If you eat this same diet and add in a lot of vegetables, your total protein calories will increase by a very small amount, as vegetables contain, on average, a few grams of protein per serving. So your total protein intake may now be 520 calories. Your total caloric intake may now be 1600 calories, as a lot of vegetables may only add a small amount to your total caloric intake as well. This new ratio, 1600/520, is also 30%. This diet, with a lot of vegetables, therefore has the same proportion of protein as the lower vegetable diet.

...Or healthy for you

Often I hear people justify these diets as healthy because along with the protein they are eating a lot of vegetables, perhaps more then they used to.

Vegetables are allowed on these diets because they are filling and the digestion of them does not yield much glucose. The whole "unintended purpose" of these diets is to stop the movement of acids into your blood. Vegetables also contain decent quantities of fiber, which helps to move acids out of your blood.

While vegetables have a small amount of fiber, are mildly alkalinizing, nutritious, and easy to digest, these benefits do not come close to offsetting the harm caused by the acidity, lack of fiber, and difficulty in digesting protein foods, particularly animal proteins like chicken, meat, and turkey.

You would be much healthier if you ate a low protein diet and very few vegetables.

If a diet calls for the restriction of carbohydrates, it is a high protein diet

If a diet calls for the reduction of bread, pasta, or other carbohydrates, it is a high protein diet. Advising someone to reduce his or her carbohydrate intake is a clever way to disguise the fact that you are advising a high protein diet. When you eat fewer carbohydrates, you greatly reduce your caloric intake so that the proportion of protein you eat increases significantly.

The Atkins diet, South Beach Diet, Weight Watchers, Zone, and numerous other diet programs are high protein diets. These diets come under many different names, but they are all the same and they all "work," as crutches, for the same reason. *Today, the vast majority of books written and advice given for weight loss and symptom reduction are high protein diets.*

Eating a lot of fish is high protein and not healthy for you

I read an article today about an actress who lost a lot of weight (in fact she now looks anorexic), and her diet was described as healthy because she eats a lot of fish and drinks a lot of red wine. Fish and red wine are highly acidic, and this is not a healthy diet.

Twenty years ago chicken was heavily promoted as a health food. Chicken cutlets were flying off the shelves. Everyone thought that if they got rid of their beef and ate a lot of chicken they would prevent heart disease and other illnesses. The outcome of these diets proved otherwise, as our health declined. The problem with the advice back then is the same with the advice given today to eat a lot of fish.

Chicken is healthier than beef, but it is not healthy to eat a lot of it. Fish is healthier than beef and chicken, but it is not healthy to eat a lot of it, either. There is a big difference between saying that something is *healthier* and saying that something is *healthy*.

Having said this, I do recommend that you replace as much of the red meat, beef, chicken, turkey, and pork that you currently eat with fish while you are healing your bowel, but I do not advertise a high fish diet as healthy, nor do I encourage the long-term consumption of it. Just as clients eventually find they lose their desire for beef, chicken, and turkey when they become healthier, they also lose their desire to eat much fish, too.

Sample diets and corresponding percentages of protein

Below are some examples of diets and an approximation of how many calories of protein they deliver.

A diet that provides excessive amounts of protein/the least healthy option, may look like this: (approximately 60% of calories from protein)

> Breakfast—2 eggs and fruit
>
> Lunch-- 6 oz. chicken, veggies
>
> Dinner—4 oz. fish, salad, veggies
>
> Snacks—4 nuts or 1 cup of yogurt or a protein shake
>
> Beverages: water, diet coke, unsweetened tea

A diet that provides more protein than is healthy, but is not as excessive as above/healthier but still unhealthy, may look like this: (approximately 40% of calories from protein)

> Breakfast—8 oz. skim milk, 10 strawberries.
>
> Lunch—6 oz. fish, ½ cup wild rice, 1 cup steamed broccoli.
>
> Dinner—4 oz. chicken, 1 flour tortilla, ½ cup vegetables.
>
> Snacks—1 orange, 9 almonds.
>
> Beverages—water, diet coke, and unsweetened tea.
>
> Other examples: Breakfast—1 ½ cups whole grain cereal, 1 cup skim milk; Lunch—1 apple, barbeque chicken pizza; Dinner—9 oz. chicken, 1 cup vegetables; Snack—1 orange, 10 pretzels.; Breakfast—scrambled eggs, whole wheat toast with peanut butter; Lunch—tuna sandwich on whole wheat bread; Dinner—chicken or fish, salad; Snack---cheese, fruit

A diet that provides adequate but not excessive amounts of protein/the healthiest option, may look like this: (approximately 10% of calories from protein)

> Breakfast—oatmeal and fruit, soymilk
>
> Lunch—bean burrito, salad
>
> Dinner—Whole grain pasta, veggies, cheese
>
> Snacks—nuts, yogurt
>
> Beverages—water, tea, fruit juice

High protein vegetarian diets aren't that high in protein

Years ago, when high protein diets began climbing in popularity, I read an article in a popular vegetarian magazine aimed at helping vegetarians achieve a high protein diet without the consumption of animal protein foods. While these diets are much healthier than diets that use animal protein—because they are much less acidic and much easier to digest—they are also generally much higher in fiber and lower in protein. For an explanation why low acid, easy-to-digest diets are healthy for you, see Chapter 9.

One serving of chicken may provide you with thirty grams of protein while one serving of beans may only contain seven, for example. This makes these diets more cleansing (more acids go into your blood), and this effect minimizes or eliminates the desirable results that one sees when eating a lot of animal protein. Not surprisingly, then, I rarely meet a client who is eating a high protein vegetarian diet and successfully treating their symptoms or weight with it. This once-popular magazine is now difficult to find.

Do not reduce your animal protein intake until your bowel is healthier!

The number one reason a client will feel worse when they start this program is because they reduce their protein intake too quickly. If after reading this you are anxious to reduce your protein intake now—don't. I am thrilled if you want to do this, but *you must be patient.*

You must create a stronger bowel before you can reduce your protein intake without feeling worse and gaining weight. Even a slight reduction of only 4-6 ounces of protein a day can stimulate your body to start cleansing before your bowel is healthy enough to handle it comfortably, and effectively.

Food Allergy, Wheat-free, Gluten-free and/or Dairy-free Crutches

This program strengthens your bowel so that dairy, wheat, and other food allergies do not exist. When you avoid a food that you are allergic to but do not heal your bowel, you may see a quick improvement in your symptoms, but you rarely see a complete elimination of them. In this program, your symptoms will be completely eliminated. When you avoid food allergens you create a stressful eating environment, with fear around food, and fear when eating out when the ingredients of a dish are not always known. When you are done with this program, you will be able to eat any food and not react, and the fear around food is eliminated.

When you avoid a food you are allergic to, you are avoiding the fact that your bowel is unhealthy, and it will continue to become less healthy even as you avoid this food, leading to more debilitating conditions down the road, including a higher possibility of early death. You are led to a false sense of security about your health. In my program, your bowel is strengthened so that not only are the allergy-triggered ear infections and eczema eliminated, but all conditions, such as weight gain, aches and pains, bloating and allergies, are also avoided.

When I was very ill, I ate a strict wheat-free, dairy-free, sugar-free diet. I followed this for approximately five years. Eventually, I just couldn't keep it up. *My symptoms improved slightly on this diet, but were still significantly worse than when I healed my bowel and body and added wheat and dairy back into my daily diet.*

These diets are more widely known about today, but this is *not* a "new" magical dietary program. Like all of the other crutches, they are back in print because there is a whole new population of people who haven't tried, and ultimately failed, following them. I have worked with many people who have failed with this approach, and some of the most seriously ill people that I have worked with have followed this approach and still remained highly symptomatic.

Food allergies and food intolerances are, physiologically, two different conditions. Neither of these would exist if your bowel was healthy, and for simplicity here, I have lumped these together and simply refer to them as allergies. Also, I focus mainly on dairy and gluten allergies as these are the most common, but this is not meant to imply that nut, egg, citrus, soy, and/or any other food allergies or intolerances are different. The concepts mentioned here apply to them too.

Gluten (wheat) and dairy are very common ingredients in the foods we eat. When these are eliminated, the majority of people replace them with high protein foods like chicken, fish, and eggs. In other words, *allergy-free diets usually turn into high protein diets, and help and hurt for the same reasons they do.*

A healthy bowel digests gluten and lactose without producing discomfort. When you focus on a strict diet and do not address your weak bowel, you may find that your symptoms improve, but as soon as you stray from the diet, they will return. And straying from this diet is very easy to do. Unfortunately, at this point, most people think they failed, rather than blame the approach. Many practitioners blame the person when they stray from this ridiculously strict diet and their symptoms return, when the real blame lies in the approach that the practitioner recommended. As in so many other cases, you have been led to believe that if something gives you immediate, short-term benefits, you are on the right track, and that the approach is not the ultimate reason for your failure.

A naturopath writes of treating a child with eczema and how the elimination of dairy produced formed stools for the first time in the child's life, and that as soon as dairy was re-introduced the symptoms returned. If a symptom returns, you have not healed your bowel or body. If you eliminate a food group and your stools improve it does not mean you have healed your bowel. You have not.

The long-term consequences of following these diets have not shown up, yet. But they will. If you do not heal your bowel and only avoid foods that you are allergic, or sensitive to, you are at risk of other serious health problems down the road. Problems like breast cancer and prostate cancer; problems that are directly associated with an unhealthy bowel.

Wheat and dairy are not the cause of your problems. They may trigger health and weight symptoms, but they are not the cause. Some people blame food allergies and intolerances on genetics. What you are not told is that yes, you can inherit an unhealthy bowel from your parents, and this will manifest as allergies and intolerances *unless you actively work to heal it.*

If your bowel were healthy you could eat these foods without feeling bad or gaining weight.

Gluten and dairy-free diets—or any other food allergy diet--do not heal your bowel.

Low Fat and Low Calorie Crutches

Low fat and low calorie diets can help you lose weight, but they too are crutches that do not heal your bowel and address the cause of your weight problems. These diets were popular prior to the low carbohydrate craze, and I have noticed food manufacturers are starting to market their foods this way again. Like high protein diets that "didn't work" when they were first introduced decades ago, neither did these. But once again, there is another enormous market of people who are overweight now that were not last time they were in vogue, and this enormous new market will buy into this philosophy like many before them. They will think this is the answer to their weight problems, until they fail, at which point they will go back to the miracle high protein diets again. This loop will go around and around and around unless people get with this program.

These diets also do nothing to strengthen your bowel, but compared to high protein diets, they are much healthier. Still, these diets are crutches and like all crutches, they ultimately fail to give you ideal health and effortless weight maintenance. Because many people will initially lose weight on them, when they fail, they will wrongly blame themselves and not the approach.

This diet is the crutch I used to maintain my thin frame for many years, before becoming extremely ill.

Alkaline "Cures" Crutches

Some books and articles claim that an alkaline diet and/or certain alkalinizing supplements will cure you of your health and weight problems. These "cures" can help you look and feel better while you heal your bowel, but I would not call them a "cure," as they treat the symptom of excess acidity in your body and not the cause, which is an unhealthy bowel that cannot efficiently eliminate acids. Alkaline foods, drinks, and supplements help buffer un-eliminated acids, reducing symptoms and weight produced by these acids, but they do not eliminate them from your body or create a bowel that can do this, and continue to do this, for you effortlessly in years to come.

Some of the more common alkaline "cures" include the ingestion of coral calcium, alkaline water, baking soda, apple cider vinegar, lemon water, and/or green drinks, like algae and wheatgrass. Some of these are more popularly promoted than others, like the apple cider vinegar "cure" which I seem to spot on the front of a magazine by the supermarket checkout at least once a year. Coral calcium was a big seller a number of years ago through a successful infomercial campaign, and lemon water has shown up on diet programs for many years. When I was very ill, I daily made an alkaline drink consisting of one cup of warm water, the juice of ½ lemon, one tablespoon of honey and one tablespoon of cider vinegar. It did not "cure" me, but I felt a little better as I was trying to figure out how to heal my body.

For most people, large amounts of the above need to be incorporated into their diet to see a difference. For example, the juice of ¼ of a lemon won't help much; squeezing the fresh juice out of four or six lemons and drinking that is more likely to.

I once had a client come see me who had been suffering with fibromyalgia. He found that ingesting a very large amount of these alkaline products noticeably eased his discomfort. His pHs were very bad however, showing a large retention of acidity in his body and organ weakness, and his bowel was eliminating very poorly. He liked his "quick fix" and didn't want to do the work of healing his bowel and body and I never saw him again. It is very difficult to maintain a daily regimen of ingesting large quantities of supplements that only "work" when you take them, and years later, it is highly likely that his symptoms have returned with a vengeance. But the most significant point of this is that even though this man felt much better on this, the acidity causing his discomfort was not eliminated. And this program did not help the condition of his bowel, either.

I had a similar experience. At one time while suffering from daily, excruciating neck pain, I took large quantities of calcium and saw a dramatic reduction in this symptom. Because I felt better, I thought I had found my cure and I focused solely on this approach for a while. A couple years later, feeling better but still not as well as I could be, I stopped the calcium and slowly my symptoms returned. My pHs were not ideal, and during the entire time I took the calcium, my bowel did not improve either.

Like all crutches, you cannot rely on these alkalinizing ones alone. In the long run, they will fail you. They are wonderful short-term crutches. Neutralizing the acids that are not being eliminated from your body will help you look and feel better, but you must heal your bowel so that your body can eliminate these acids from your body in the first place, as well as in the long-term. If you have holes in your trash can and trash leaks out, it will be helpful to spray that trash with perfume so that it doesn't smell, but this does nothing to fix the holes in the trashcan that allowed it to leak out in the first place. And these holes will eventually cause your trashcan to fall apart. The perfume does not prevent this from happening. Your bowel bacteria need to be fixed so that acids can be eliminated. Then you don't have to rely on alkalinizing supplements and diets to neutralize them. Also, your bowel bacteria do more than just eliminate acids, as described in Chapter 4, and ignoring this will lead to serious trouble down the road.

Alkaline diets and cures can help you lose weight and feel better. They are generally not dangerous like many other weight loss and drug crutches, and I encourage you to utilize these approaches while healing your bowel and body.

Macrobiotic Crutches

When I became ill these diets were popular and I read a lot about them. This information was part of the foundation upon which this program evolved. Early on I even called my dietary advice "American Macrobiotics." To simplify, macrobiotics promotes the consumption of a balance of yin and yang foods. Because these terms were unfamiliar to my clients and because many Asian foods were as well, I taught these concepts using terms and food that my clients could connect with. Acid and alkaline food choices, which are described further in Chapter 9, are a mirror of yin and yang ones. The ultimate objective and outcome is the same.

Just the other day I heard that these diets were gaining popularity again in Hollywood. I am thrilled, as this implies that people are beginning to lose interest in the harmful high protein diets, but I am skeptical that this will last long. I suspect that like all other "diets" that have come and gone and resurfaced, this one too will meet that fate.

Compared to high protein diets, a macrobiotic one is much healthier. Again, it is essentially the same diet that I promote and label a pH balanced diet. It is generally a high fiber, high carbohydrate, alkalinizing diet, although I have seen it followed where it becomes another high protein diet. It doesn't matter what you call a high protein diet. The name does not change the fact that it is harmful.

A properly balanced macrobiotic or pH balanced diet is healthy, but it is very difficult to maintain, especially when your bowel is weak. It also does nothing to heal your bowel. Unlike a high protein diet that makes your bowel less healthy, this diet does not, but it does not fix it, either. A macrobiotic diet is a healthy crutch to use while you heal your bowel, but if you try it without healing your bowel, your ultimate failure rate with it will be very high. This book promotes a pH balanced diet, but the heart of healing and achieving a long, happy, healthy life requires a healthy bowel.

Cleansing and Fasting Crutches

Every spring, cleansing programs and fasts are promoted in health food stores and alternative health publications. They promise to help one lose weight, feel better, and eliminate accumulated toxins/acids in anywhere from three days to two weeks. Some temporary weight loss or symptom reduction may occur, but this is short lived, and frequent cleanses or fasts to repeat this result are not necessarily safe or desirable. The dependence on a cleanse or fast to produce results means that you are avoiding the weakness in your bowel that caused your health and weight problems in the first place. Think of a cleanse or fast as emptying your trashcans for one day. *A cleanse or fast will not heal your bowel bacteria and it would take numerous ones, over many years, before the majority of old, accumulated acidity in your body were eliminated.*

The promise of toxin or acid elimination is highly over-exaggerated and misleading. During a cleansing diet, a very small amount of stored up toxins in your cells and fat cells may be moved into your bloodstream, but this is uncomfortable and worse, unproductive, if they cannot be eliminated. A healthy bowel is needed to eliminate this waste, and since most people have an unhealthy one, this is not accomplished. *Un-eliminated toxins go right back to where they came from.*

During some cleanses or fasts, you may lose weight, but it has nothing to do with a significant elimination of toxins or improvement in your health. During a cleanse, your caloric intake is greatly reduced, and this generally results in temporary weight loss, whatever name you call it! Because one cleanse does not create a healthier body—one that would allow you to lose weight and keep it off—the weight you do lose during this cleanse will eventually return. Often this happens within one week of stopping it.

Most of the improvement in your symptoms that you feel during these programs is due to that fact that during this time "hardly any rain hits the roof." In other words, your body is not made much stronger or healthier— the holes are not fixed—there is simply less stress placed on it, and you feel better because of it. These cleanses eliminate stressful, acidic foods like sugar and coffee and alcohol, and people usually feel or look better when this "rain" is eliminated. Some cleanses incorporate alkaline foods like lemon juice and maple syrup which buffer acids, but do not eliminate them. When you stop the cleanse and go back to your usual diet, however, any symptoms that went away will often quickly return.

When I was very ill I did many fasts and cleanses and during them much of the pain and inflammation I had went away. As soon as I stopped the cleanse, the pain returned at the same level that it was before the cleanse. After doing numerous cleanses, I still had an enormous amount of toxicity in my body. I have a client who came to see me after ten years of rigorous fasting. Her experience included long fasts of ten days or more. Yet when she entered my office, a significant amount of toxins were still stored in her body. This client also came in with an unhealthy bowel. All of those years of fasting did not heal it.

In some cases, fasts and cleanses can be dangerous. I met a woman twenty years ago who had gone to a cleansing center and became very dehydrated. Fortunately, someone at the center recognized this and helped to remedy it, but is this ok? Also, here she was, years later, still battling with health and weight problems.

Sometimes when you cleanse your body, acids are stirred up and sent into your organs of elimination to be eliminated. Excess un-eliminated acidity can cause electrolyte imbalances and dehydration. This is not safe. This reaction does not occur on this program. In this program, your bowel is healed before any cleansing takes place. This way, when acids are released into your blood and sent into your organs of elimination, your bowel efficiently eliminates them, your kidneys are not stressed, and dehydration does not occur.

If you do a cleanse and your stools become loose, it is a sign that you need to stop the cleanse because the toxins are not getting eliminated, and you may not only become dehydrated, but these toxins will just get reabsorbed, anyway. I have unfortunately read about cleanses where loose stools or diarrhea are considered a healing reaction and not respected as the danger that they are. If you cleanse and your bowels get loose, not only should this be your signal to stop, it should alert you of the necessity to heal the bacterial environment in your bowel. This is an important signal your body is giving you, and you would be wise to respect it.

The greatest value of these programs is that they get you thinking about toxins. They also give you an opportunity to see and feel your health potential. You get to see that there is an answer to your problems that perhaps, up until then, you were told were only treatable with drugs, or nothing at all. This was true for me. When my excruciating pain disappeared during a fast, I knew that my body could feel dramatically different. It kept my hopes up and me fighting for the answer, which I eventually found.

If you want to incorporate a cleansing diet into this program, that is fine. Just make sure that you do it safely. There are numerous books and other references that can help you with this. Keep in perspective the limitations of what you are accomplishing during this. And if you find any of these cleanses too difficult, don't worry. None of these are necessary for you to achieve supreme health and permanent weight loss on this program.

In fact, this program guides you to a way of eating and living that incorporates what you might call "mini-fasts." This is much more valuable than occasional, longer-term fasting. By eating an easier to digest diet, increasing your fiber and water intake, lowering salt consumption, sweating and deep breathing, you increase the daily elimination of toxins and fat from your body. *More importantly, by improving the function of your bowel—which fasting alone does not do—you are creating a healthy system that will naturally eliminate these toxins for you-- steadily, rapidly, safely, and permanently.*

If done wisely—i.e. the fast or cleanse is stopped if diarrhea or loose bowels occurs—a fast or cleanse is less harmful than drugs or a high protein diet as a means of treating symptoms and losing weight while you heal your bowel and body.

Raw Food Crutches

I first read about raw food diets twenty years ago. The idea is to eat only raw, uncooked foods, as they are very easy to digest, cleansing, and contain enzymes that help your body heal. Of all the programs I tried, I never did this one. I ate a lot of raw, sprouted, fermented, cultured, and other enzyme-rich foods, but I never ate only these. By the time I read about these diets I was burned out from all of my rigid diets and was focused on healing my bowel. I also thought about the long-living Asians who eat a lot of cooked foods, so this diet just didn't seem like the answer for me. I have met others who have eaten this way, however, and I know from my extensive experience in healing the bowel and body, the advantages and disadvantages of this approach.

The advantage of eating a raw food diet is that it is healthy for you. These foods are low in acidity, easy to digest, and high in fiber; all qualifications that lend to helping create a healthy body. People who eat these diets tend to lose weight and can also feel better, partly because these are low calorie diets that contain no highly acidic foods that can trigger symptoms. These diets are cleansing and help move acids from your cells and blood into your bowel. They are particularly valuable for people with degenerative diseases like cancer and heart disease. Compared to low carbohydrate and/or low calorie diets, they are much healthier for you.

On the flip side, these diets are rigid and extremely difficult to follow. They breed fear and social isolation, and this is not healthy for you. The fear of eating cooked food, because cooking destroys all enzymes and some nutrients in the food, is unjustified. A healthy bowel produces healing and digestive enzymes for you. When your bowel is healthy, you don't need to rely on raw foods for these enzymes. I have worked with people who have followed these diets who presented themselves to me with health conditions and unhealthy bowels. These diets help move acids into your bowel, but they do not heal your bowel. In fact, because these diets are very high in fiber and move a lot of acidity into your bowel, they can trigger a great amount of intestinal discomfort, gas, bloating, diarrhea, and other problems that can cause one to easily abandon this approach. It also means, once again, that toxins are *not* being eliminated and you are *not* healing your body, as proponents of these claim. Professionally, I do not recommend them.

Raw food diets are crutches, and if you have to eat this way all the time to keep your blood sugar stable, for example, you haven't really "reversed" your diabetes, as proponents of these claim. When you heal your bowel, you will be able to eat cooked foods, even sugar, without your blood sugar going out of balance!

Raw food diets have value but do not heal your bowel, and if you heal your bowel, you will attain a much higher level of health than if you only follow this diet. A healthy bowel and body will stay that way, even if cooked foods are consumed.

My Experience with Dietary Crutches

You will want less animal protein too

Growing up, I didn't eat much food. When I did eat, the foods I loved most were steak, meat, sugar, eggs, and refined carbohydrates like bagels and pizza. When I became very ill I was put on a high protein diet. Because my organs were already very unhealthy, it didn't take very long for my symptoms and health to noticeably degenerate. I followed the diet for about nine months and ended up sicker than ever.

When I healed my bowel and body my interest in animal protein was eliminated. For many years now I have eaten a mostly vegetarian diet. When I eat animal protein, it is due to convenience or a desire for more variety in my diet, but after I eat it, I find myself wanting it even less, not more. My muscle tone is much more defined now, as a vegetarian, than it was when I ate a lot of meat. I was a vegetarian throughout my pregnancy and I had no problems during it. I had no anemia, no water retention, no nausea, and no complications during the births of my children at home. My children have always eaten a diet considered low in protein by modern standards, but they are strong, well built, and healthy.

In all of the years that I have worked as a nutritionist, I have consistently advised an eventual low protein diet. This will never change. In the same period, the medical profession, diet promoters, and even many natural health practitioners have changed their dietary advice a number of times, particularly in regards to protein intake. As long as people keep focusing on treating their symptoms and do not heal their bowels, the dietary contradictions will continue. When they start to focus on good health, there will be no confusion.

My clients always find that as their bowel becomes healthier and they become healthier, their desire for protein goes down. It never goes up, regardless of their blood type or any other variable that is used to justify a higher intake.

While you are healing your bowel and body there are some safe and healthy dietary crutches that you can adopt to help you look and feel better. For more information on these refer to Chapter 9.

Chapter Six

A Healthy Bowel Explained

The health of your bowel is not simply determined by the frequency and form of your stools.

The form of your stools is much more important than the frequency of your elimination.

Your stools should be frequent and well-formed regardless of what you eat.

Misunderstandings about bowel function are a top reason why people fail to heal their bowel and body.

Optimum Elimination (Teenagers and Adults)

The description of optimum bowel function can be broken down into two categories: **frequency, and form of your stools.**

Frequency

Healthy elimination occurs approximately two times a day. The majority should occur prior to noon, however, it is more important that the frequency exists, than that it is at a particular time of the day. To determine an accurate reading of frequency you must include all of the times that you eliminate, even if only a very small piece of stool comes out. Also, you need to count the times that you go as separate even if they occur only one hour after the previous bowel movement. **Going more than three times a day is worse than going once every other day.**

More importantly, the form

Good form to your stools is much more important than good frequency. The better the form is, the more acids that you are eliminating. The better the form is, the better you will look and feel. If your stools are well-formed

you will automatically have good frequency; good frequency, however, does not automatically ensure good form.

Your stools should be one to one and a half inches around. You do not need to measure them, but get out a ruler and see how large this is in diameter, and then look at your stools to see if they are too skinny or too wide. Most of my clients have stools that are too skinny when they start this program. You are eliminating more acids when they are too wide than when they are too skinny.

Your stools should be easy to pass. Urgent elimination is worse than the need to strain. If you have a history of hemorrhoids or fissures the idea of having to strain may concern you, but healing your bowel will eliminate these problems, not create them. Straining does not cause hemorrhoids and fissures; excess unformed acids in your bowel that irritate the tissues and trigger inflammation cause them. The better formed your stools are, the fewer unformed acids and the fewer of these problems you will have.

Your stools should be smooth and firm, like a peeled banana. Hard, lumpy stools are better than flakey, raggedy, airy, mushy, or loose stools. They should not explode when you flush the toilet.

Each time you eliminate there should be two to three pieces of stool that are each four to six inches in length. Having one long stool is better than having a number of shorter ones.

You should have no gas or bloating, regardless of what you eat, even if you eat foods like cabbage, beans, or broccoli. Gas is caused by the poor breakdown of the insoluble fibers in your diet or difficulty digesting lactose, the sugar in milk, which happens when your bowel bacterial environment is unhealthy. Gas is also created in response to unformed acids.

The color of your stools should be medium brown. Light brown, black, clay colored, green, and orange stools are all signs of poor elimination.

Your stools should be semi-floating, like a submarine. It is better if your stools sink to the bottom of the toilet than if they float on top of the surface of the water. As your bowel becomes healthier, this is one of the last variables to change.

There should be no odor to your stools. As this improves you may find that you are more comfortable eliminating in public places.

There should be no undigested food in your stools like corn kernels, seeds, or tomato skins. When your bowel bacterial environment is unhealthy, fibrous foods like these are not completely digested, hence the appearance of them in your stool.

After eliminating, only one wipe with the toilet paper should be needed to be clean. When your stools are really loose often only one wipe is needed, but obviously the form of your stool is terrible anyway.

In summary, optimum elimination of a teenager/adult has the following characteristics

Frequency

1. 2x/day--- better less than 1x/day than more than 3x/day

2. Most elimination should occur in the morning before noon

Form

1. About 1 to 1 ½ inches in diameter--- better too wide than too skinny

2. Easy to pass--- straining better than urgency

3. Firm, well-formed, smooth texture—better too hard then soft, mushy, or flakey

4. Sufficient quantity-- 2-3 pieces, 4-6 inches in length—better too long than too short

5. No gas or bloating, regardless of what you eat

6. Medium brown in color

7. Semi-floating—better sinking than floating

8. No odor

9. No undigested food

10. One wipe

Optimum Elimination (Children and Babies)

The normal, healthy bowel function for a baby up to two to three months old is frequent and loose. A breast-fed baby should have a very yellowy stool. Formula fed babies will have less frequent and darker stools than a breast-fed baby. Breast milk has an ingredient unlike formula that has a laxative effect. This is desirable, as it is helpful and healthy for your baby to be given "extra help" in the first couple months of life in eliminating any toxins accumulated while in the womb. A healthy bowel bacterial environment is needed for proper elimination, but this has not yet been established in your newborn, hence the "need for" this laxative. The design of the human body is simply spectacular.

At two to three months old, your baby's stools should begin to slow down and firm up. By age three to four months, they should not be eliminating more than two to three times a day. At this age, the stools should have a sticky consistency, somewhat like peanut butter. Because your baby is eliminating in a diaper the stool will not appear formed in it. A formed or hard stool is not healthy, nor is one that is liquid. Their stools should be brown and never green or any other color.

The stools of a young child, approximately age three to thirteen, should be just like those of an adult, only thinner. The ideal diameter of a stool is a product of the diameter of the bowel, and a young child has a smaller and skinnier bowel than an adult. The ideal diameter of a child's stool is closer to ½ - 1 inch around. For a baby or young child, it is still relevant to observe the frequency of his stools, the color, existence of gas, odor, and/or undigested food to get an idea of how healthy his or her elimination is.

I am mortified every time I hear a pediatrician has told a mom that their baby's infrequent elimination is nothing to worry about. While I too would say don't worry, it is not a sign of eminent danger, it is definitely something to be concerned about, and action should be taken now to help heal their bowel. Some doctors will say that is normal for babies to poop often or rarely. This is true, but then again, it is normal for babies and children in this country to experience frequent colds, fevers, ear infections, asthma, eczema, asthma, and ADD.

So, is this what you want for your child, or would you like something a lot different and better than "normal?" A child who eliminates healthfully will rarely experience these problems, if at all.

Stool definitions that need to be clarified

The above descriptions of the ideal frequency and form of elimination are given to my clients on the first day that we begin this program together. It is vital that we are both "on the same page" when discussing this. Even with these specific guidelines, some clients provide me with bowel descriptions that are inaccurate. For example, I have had clients tell me that their elimination was fantastic, only to question further and discover that, more accurately, their elimination is fantastic *compared to what it used to be*, not compared to the description given above.

As much as possible, try to use the descriptions I have outlined above. This will help you heal your bowel and body much more quickly as you get into the actual healing work presented in the next chapter. They will help guide you in knowing how many of the bowel-healing products, that are discussed in the next chapter, you should take in order to accomplish this. If you heal too slow or too fast, you will fail to heal at all. Additionally, make sure that you use the following descriptions and not your own.

Constipation— there are two commonly used definitions for constipation. In the first, constipation is defined as infrequent bowel movements that are less than once a day. In the second, bowel movements are daily, but the elimination of the stool requires straining and effort. Some clients also describe constipation as stools that are small and hard. For the sake of clarity here, if I refer to constipation, I am referring to infrequent bowel movements.

Diarrhea—this is defined as a watery stool.

Loose stools—the stools are considered loose if they are mushy, flakey, soft piles, or are formed stools that disintegrate upon flushing the toilet.

How Stools Are Formed

Frequent elimination with poor form is the least healthy and most inefficient elimination pattern and leads to the greatest health and weight problems. Unfortunately, the frequency of your bowel movements is the variable that is most talked about in this country. The form of your stools, which is the variable that is far more significant, is rarely discussed, and people have a very limited awareness of the harm poorly formed stools create on their health and weight. Even the wonderful books written many years ago on bowel health emphasized the frequency of elimination, and today little has changed.

In order to understand why this is so, how to heal your bowel, and to reduce the misunderstandings that lead to failure, you must understand how a stool is formed in the first place, and the conditions that create loose stools, infrequent stools, and ideal elimination.

The frequency and form of your stools is determined by two variables: the health of the bacteria in your bowel, and the quantity of acidity, or toxins, in it. One of the jobs of your bowel bacteria is to convert acids into stools. If your trashcan has a lot of holes in it, the trash will leak out all over the front yard and make a mess. In this analogy, a poor bacterial environment causes the holes. *The more trash that leaks out, the worse your bowel movements are.*

On the other hand, if your trashcan has no holes but simply more trash in it than it can handle, trash will again leak out on the front yard and you will have poor bowel movements.

Finally, if you never throw trash into your trashcan, whether it has holes in it or not, there will be no trash to eliminate when the trash man comes. If there is not much waste, or acids, in your bowel, your bowel movements can be slow due to the lack of acids to eliminate.

The frequency of your elimination is also influenced by an action called peristalsis. Peristalsis refers to the contraction of the bowel muscle. This contraction squeezes the contents in the bowel out of your body. Peristalsis occurs automatically in the morning and results in a gentle contraction of your bowel.

Below are general descriptions of three different states of elimination. This does not cover all of the possibilities but is intended to help you have a better understanding of how your bowel works, and with that, a better understanding of how to heal it.

Worst elimination: frequent but not well-formed

The worst elimination occurs when you have frequent bowel movements of one or more times a day and your stools are poorly formed. Because of a very weak intestinal environment and/or an enormous amount of excess acidity in your bowel, very little of this acidity is converted into a stool. Most of the trash in your trashcan is not contained in a trash bag and it leaks out of it.

In this scenario, *a lot of these acids* get reabsorbed into your lymph and blood, where they cause symptoms, nutrient deficiencies, water retention, fat production, weight gain, and illness.

The presence of many unformed acids causes your body to go into crisis mode. This excess acidity is irritating and damaging to your bowel. To protect itself, your bowel will be stimulated to contract more frequently and intensely in an attempt to eliminate these unformed acids. This results in frequent bowel movements of one or more times a day.

Water is also pulled from your cells and into your bowel in an attempt to dilute the acidity so that harm to the cells of your bowel is minimized. This can lead to dehydration and electrolyte imbalances, both of which are harmful to the health of the rest of your body. If a large amount of extra water is needed to dilute these acids, your stools will become mushy or loose. If a smaller amount of acidity is in your bowel then smaller amounts of water are flushed into it, and this can cause your stools to appear skinny, soft, flakey, and semi-loose. Your stools can also appear too short or small and hard, reflecting the fact that only a small amount of the acidity was converted into a stool. Unformed acids in your bowel cause gas and bloating, and they feed Candida, yeast, bad bacteria, and other unwanted organisms.

Better elimination: infrequent but better form

Better elimination occurs when there are infrequent bowel movements— possibly five to seven times a week—and better form than above, but still less than ideal. Better form is defined as larger, longer, less flakey and firmer stools. In this scenario, acids are still reabsorbed into your body, but much less so than in the worst-case scenario above, resulting in less weight gain and fewer symptoms and illness.

In this case, more of the acids in your bowel have been turned into stool than in the first case above. A healthier bowel bacterial environment and/or fewer acids in it, cause your stools to be better formed. Fewer unformed acids also mean less gas. Still, your bowel environment is not perfectly healthy and/or there is more acidity than it can handle, so only some of it is formed into stools, not all of it. This creates a stool that is larger than in the first case, but still not large enough to be eliminated quickly and efficiently when peristalsis occurs. If your stool is not large enough, it will not be squeezed out easily.

Because more acids are absorbed and turned into a stool, there are less unformed acids than in the case above and this eliminates the "crisis reaction" In other words, because your bowel is not as stressed out and threatened, your body does not need to move extra water into it, and it is not stimulated to contract more intensely as above. Your stool, however, is not large enough to come out one day and often will come out the next, as it becomes larger (as it sits in your colon and more acids are formed up.) This produces a stool that tends to be too large, long, and/or harder. This scenario also results in less gas and less Candida, yeast, and other similar problems, as there are fewer unformed acids to trigger these.

Best elimination: good frequency and form

The best elimination occurs when you eliminate about two times a day and your stools are perfectly formed. When the bacterial environment in your bowel is healthy and there is not an excess of acidity in it, all of the acids in it are efficiently turned into stools. There are no leftover acids to be reabsorbed into your body causing symptoms, illness and weight gain. There are no extra acids to cause looseness or gas either. This well-formed stool is large enough to be quickly and easily eliminated when your bowel contracts.

Frequent elimination is only healthy and beneficial to your health and weight if your stools are very well-formed, as described above.

As you heal, form improves before frequency

Your bowel will not and cannot heal overnight! It will take some time before it is stronger and better form and frequency is seen. The earlier description of ideal bowel health is not something that will occur immediately, but rather it is a destination that you will be driving towards.

There is a process and progression of change that occurs during the healing of your bowel that is often misunderstood by those on the right path with the wrong information about what to expect. The fewer misunderstandings you have, the quicker you will heal your bowel and reach your health and weight potential.

As your bowel health improves, the form will continuously improve as well. If you currently have frequent but poorly formed stools, the frequency, however, will slow down as your bowel becomes healthier and your stools become better formed. Only later, when your bowel has become much healthier, will you have frequent *and* well-formed stools.

In other words, in referring to the above description of how stools are formed, if you start with the worst elimination, you must proceed to better elimination before you get to the best elimination. If you are in California at the start of this program you must drive through Ohio to get to Nantucket, and in Ohio, your bowel movements will be slower, but better formed. You cannot fly over Ohio. Not when you heal.

If you reach this stage you will move out of it, as long as you continue with healing your bowel. If you reach Ohio you will not get stuck there if you keep driving the car. Moving out of this stage takes you to a state of elimination that is usually once a day and stools that are always formed, albeit perhaps a bit too wide or long or hard. Even though this is not yet ideal, it is far superior to the elimination of the vast majority of people. Keep driving the car and eventually you will get to the ideal elimination. Keep healing your bowel and eventually it will be healthy enough to produce the ideal elimination for you.

It is much healthier, and you are eliminating more acidity, if you go every other day and your stool is wide and hard then if you go every day and your stools are skinny or too short. I get phone calls from clients frequently when they reach this less frequent stage, even though I have explained beforehand that it will occur, that it is positive, and it won't last forever. When this happens, clients look and feel better than before starting this program, but they tend to experience some mental anguish and concern. Just today a client informed me that when she took the products I suggested to immediately help form up the acids in her bowel (this is discussed in Chapter 8), her bowel movements became slower and harder, but her daily migraines were not occurring.

Infrequent elimination evokes a state of fear and mental discomfort. Ironically, the true fear should occur when there are frequent but poorly formed stools, as this is the most dangerous elimination, but we have not been conditioned to be fearful of it. *This misplaced fear is a significant reason for the failure of people to heal their bowel and body.*

The healing of your bowel will follow the guideline below

Worst------------------------Better------------------------Best

2x/day or >, "0" form*   0-1x/day, "5" form   2x/day, "10" form

*If using a scale to rate the overall form of your stools, a "1" indicates the worst form and a "10" indicates the best.

Description of a Healthy Bowel

The description of ideal bowel movements given earlier provides one way for you to determine if your bowel is healthy. If you do not meet all of the above criteria, then your bowel is not healthy. However, things are not that simple or conclusive. It is possible to meet most of these criteria and still have a very unhealthy bowel.

The frequency and form of your stools should meet the ideal bowel description criteria all of the time, regardless of what you eat. If your stools are normally well-formed but become looser under stress, during your period, or when you eat spicy foods, more fruit or more carbohydrates—your bowel is not as healthy as it could be.

When your bowel is healthy, a low protein diet will not cause problems with the frequency or form of your stools. When your bowel is healthy you will be able to eat only vegetables and carbohydrates some days and still maintain ideal bowel movements.

A healthy bowel will tolerate a high fiber diet without producing gas, looseness, or discomfort.

A healthy bowel will reject the products used to improve the bacterial environment as instructed in the next chapter on healing your bowel. A healthy bacterial environment in your bowel will produce loose stools if these products are taken; the lack of loose stools after taking these products confirms a bowel weakness. Just one *Bowel Strength* a day and/or one billion organisms of acidophilus a day should be too strong and produce loose stools. These products are used for healing your bowel bacterial environment and are discussed in length in Chapter 7. If you take these products and they do not cause gas or loose stools, your bowel is not as healthy as it could be. **The more of these supplements that you can tolerate, the weaker your bowel is, the more dangerous the situation is, and the more important it is that you aggressively heal it now.**

The existence of gluten allergies, lactose allergies, hemorrhoids, diverticulitis, polyps, appendicitis, ulcers, Chron's, celiac, colitis, colon cancer, or any other bowel disease or condition are signs that your bowel is extremely weak and unhealthy. If you do not currently have one of these conditions it does not mean that your bowel is healthy, and if you ignore an unhealthy bowel for many years, you have a much greater chance of eventually reaching these states than if you don't ignore it.

Your bowel movements can be good even if your bowel is unhealthy

Sometimes a new client will say to me, "My stools are pretty well-formed but I am still overweight, or I still have symptoms, or a disease. Does that mean that for me, an unhealthy bowel has nothing to do with my problems? Does it mean there is no hope for me? Does it mean that your program doesn't work for everyone?" The answer to these questions is an emphatic no!

The form and frequency of your elimination by itself does not guarantee that your bowel is healthy. If there are a lot of holes in the trashcan but you don't throw much trash into it, your yard won't get too messy. If your bowel bacterial environment is unhealthy but few acids are going into your bowel, your stools may be pretty good.

There are two main reasons why very little acidity could be entering your bowel. One, a high protein diet—which many of you eat—slows down the cleansing of your organs and subsequent movement of acids into your bowel. If you eat a high protein diet your stools will be different than if you don't, and they will not accurately reflect the true health of your bowel. People eating this type of diet can easily be fooled into believing that their bowel is much healthier than it really is. **Because so many people are now following low carbohydrate, low-cleansing diets, many people dangerously believe that their bowels are healthier than they really are too.**

Two, your organs must be healthy and strong to move acids from your body into your bowel. If they are not, very little acidity may be reaching it.

You can test the true health of your bowel by eating a highly acidic, high carbohydrate, cleansing diet for a few days. Eat only pizza, sugar, coffee, peaches, and spicy foods for three days, and if you experience gas, bloating, constipation and/or mushier stools, your bowel is unhealthy.

Recently a client came to see me who at the age of 40 was dealing with re-occurring colon cancer that had spread. He had a history of eating a high protein diet. He presented himself to me with frequent, well-formed stools. You cannot have colon cancer and a healthy bowel! Sure enough, once I had him completely stop eating high protein foods and switch to a more cleansing diet, one that causes acids to move into the bowel, he began to have diarrhea. Doing this exposed the weakness in his bowel.

I have worked with many clients who have come in with all kinds of health and weight problems, and if at first their bowel movements aren't too bad, we always discover that their bowel is unhealthy.

Then again, your bowel may be healthier than you think

On the other hand, if there are only a few holes in your trashcan but a lot of trash going into it, your yard will be a mess. If your bowel bacteria are only somewhat unhealthy but you eat a very cleansing, high fiber, low protein diet, your stools can be bad, and you may think that you are less healthy than you really are. If you are in this situation, you will benefit greatly from healing your bowel. The point is, bowel health cannot simply be determined by the quality of your bowel movements. When I see a client and try to estimate the health of their bowel, I take in consideration how cleansing their diet is as well as their symptoms, but **ultimately, the most accurate test of your bowel health is your tolerance to the bowel healing products, as described in Chapter 7.**

I have yet to work with someone who has a healthy bowel when they come into my office, and I have yet to work with someone who doesn't feel and look better once their elimination improves. I am positive that all of you reading this book, who work hard to maintain your weight or have symptoms, addictions, or an illness, have an unhealthy bowel. Never once over the years have you been told how to fix your bowel. This book will teach you how.

A good colonoscopy does not mean your bowel is healthy

A lack of polyps or cancer detected during a colonoscopy does not mean your colon, or bowel, is healthy. If you suffer from Irritable Bowel Syndrome (IBS), a colonoscopy will not show any bleeding or disease, either. *A colonoscopy cannot measure the intestinal bacterial health of your bowel.*

If non-cancerous polyps are found, having them removed is a good idea, but ignoring them is not. This is a red flag that your bowel is very unhealthy and if you simply remove the polyps but do not heal your bowel, something more serious will occur later on.

Stool analysis tests are a waste of money

Some practitioners send stool samples to labs to have them tested for bacterial levels, parasites, Candida, and other imbalances and problems. These tests can cost up to $500 and are a waste of your hard earned money. Practitioners who do not specialize in healing the bowel order these tests; they specialize in treating symptoms, and people who do, tend to love lab tests. If you are told you need to have one of these done in order to assess the health of your bowel, find someone else to help you.

Like all laboratory tests, stool analysis tests are inaccurate and are not a good measurement of the health of your bowel. The fact that some practitioners need these in order to determine if your bowel is unhealthy astounds me. It is extremely easy to figure this out. The guidelines I provided you with above are all you need to make this determination.

I have focused on healing the bowel of every client I have seen for the last sixteen years. I do not know of any acupuncturist, chiropractor, naturopath, or doctor who has done the same. I have helped numerous people heal their bowel and body, and I have never ordered a stool analysis. Like blood tests, they can do more harm than good, as things can like look better or worse than they really are.

Many years ago I had a client who had horrible bowel problems and he wanted a stool test done because he didn't want to believe that his bowel was very unhealthy. Another practitioner ordered it for him and it came back showing that his bowel was healthy. I told him that was impossible and we scheduled a phone conference with a doctor at the lab, which was a very popular stool analysis lab in North Carolina, who told us that the results were not conclusive because many stool analyses would need to be done over a week's time to really comprehend what was going on. In other words, he, and others who used this lab, spent $500 for a test whose results could not even be guaranteed as valid.

If you need a laboratory or medical test to confirm that your bowel is unhealthy, then you are not ready to heal your body. Trying to prove that you are healthier than you really are, which is the attitude I find most prevalent among people who want a test, rather than directing this energy into healing your body, will eventually be very dangerous to your health and livelihood.

I am not aware of any laboratory test in this country that can accurately determine bowel health.

More Bowel Misunderstandings

A lifetime of bad stools does not guarantee a future of them

Many people ask, "I have had infrequent bowel movements my entire life so isn't that my personal ideal elimination. How can it be different if it has always been that way?"

Just because you were born with ten toes and ten fingers does not mean that you were born with a perfectly healthy bowel. Do not limit yourself by what you think is normal. If your house was originally built with cheap windows, you can replace them with better quality ones. My bowel movements were horrible all of my life until I healed my bowel, and many clients have also seen their bowel movements become better than ever as they healed it.

What you eat is not what comes out

Clients often try to justify their low output of waste as a product of having not eaten much the day before. **If you eat very little food one day, you should still have a healthy elimination with good quantity, form, and frequency.**

Most of the contents of your stools are the product of bulk-forming fiber and the fermentation of acids, not food, into stool by your intestinal bacteria. Acids comprise most of the waste that needs to be eliminated daily. Your body should use the majority of the food you eat. It should be turned into energy and new cells, for example, and there should be a relatively small amount of waste leftover that your bowel needs to eliminate. (Think about what happens when you eat a loaf of bread. The bread is eaten and only a small plastic package is left to throw into your trashcan.) This happens when you eat a low acid, easy to digest diet, as taught in this program. These foods create a lot more good material for your body and a lot less waste than hard to digest, highly acidic diets, like high protein diets. Processed foods that contain a lot of preservatives and food colorings—items that are not converted into energy or new cells by your body—create more waste that needs to be eliminated. You likely have a vast accumulation of old acidity in your body that needs to be eliminated as well. Pollutants and other environmental toxins inhaled during the day, as well as old cells that have been replaced with new ones, creates ample waste that needs to be eliminated daily.

An unhealthy bowel causes constipation, diarrhea, and other problems.

Constipation is not caused by a lack of exercise, water, fiber, or changes in your routine. An unhealthy bowel causes it. If your bowel is unhealthy, these items can trigger constipation, but they are not the cause.

Likewise, stress, dairy products, or spicy foods do not cause diarrhea. An unhealthy bowel causes it, too. If your bowel is unhealthy, these items can trigger diarrhea, but they are not the cause.

Variations in your stools are due to variations in the amount of acidity in your bowel

You may find that on some days your stools are mushy and other days they are hard. What does this mean? The weakness in your bowel bacteria, or the holes in your trashcan, does not vary from day to day, but the amount of acidity, or trash, going into it can. Remember, the quality and frequency of your stools reflects both the bacterial environment in your bowel *and* the amount of acidity in it. If your stools are mushy one day and slow and hard the next, on the day they were hard there was less acidity in your bowel than on the day they were mushy.

The less healthy your bowel is, the more variable your elimination can be. The healthier your bowel, the less variation you will have. The fewer holes in your roof, the more it can rain before your house gets wet. Most importantly here is the fact that it is not the health of your bowel that is changing day to day, and that the health of your bowel cannot be changed, or improved, in one day either.

Elimination after every meal is not ideal

Some people who give bowel advice say, "if you eat three meals a day and only eliminate once a day, you are storing the other two meals." They also claim that you should eliminate after every meal, because babies do, and the assumption is made that this should apply to adults as well. This is entirely wrong. Another so-called expert says that a new baby eliminates after every meal because they have not had a chance for toxins to accumulate. This is wrong too.

A baby's intestinal system is unique for a unique time of life. It reflects the amazing design of the human body. A baby also sleeps 12-16 hours a day, but that does not mean that as older children or adults we too need that much sleep. Breast-fed babies poop a lot because breast milk has a laxative effect. Given that the form of the stool is greatly undervalued and misunderstood, and that most people eliminate frequently but with poorly formed stools, I believe that some people who advise that your bowel moves after every meal are themselves dealing with an unhealthy intestinal environment and as a result, have frequent, poorly formed stools. Perhaps they want to believe they are healthier than they really are and use this "babies poop after every meal" explanation as a way to justify their own elimination pattern. A healthy bowel will not eliminate after every meal. The majority of the elimination will occur in the morning before noon.

More definitions and confusion about constipation

Healing your bowel will not produce very infrequent bowel movements, or bowels that move only every three days or longer. If your bowel movements are one or more times a day and not well-formed when you start this program, they will become slower and better formed as you heal, as described earlier, but they will not become very infrequent. You will not miss more than one day in a row of elimination. (Exception: this can occur if you currently rely on laxatives to have a bowel movement—like magnesium, senna, vitamin C, aloe or cascara---and you stop these before you heal your bowel. If you do, blame this, and not the bowel-healing supplements, for your constipation.)

Frequent bowel movements depend in part on the contraction, or peristalsis, of your bowel. This is an automatic reaction that occurs daily. A few scenarios can cause this peristalsis to be hampered, causing very infrequent bowel movements.

Constipation from muscle relaxants and illness

Muscle relaxants reduce the contraction of all muscles in your body, including your bowel. These are commonly prescribed after surgery and for aches and pains. In cases of a serious illness and very poor health, peristalsis can be hampered because of the general inability of your body to function properly. In these situations you may find that your bowel movements become less frequent. In these situations, a natural laxative may be used, stopping this if your bowels become more than once a day and loosely formed.

Traveler's constipation

According to Dr. Oz, forty-two million Americans suffer from traveler's constipation. He attributes this to a variety of variables, including an increase in stress and inability to relax the muscles in the bowel due to "strange toilet syndrome," less water and fiber, and a disturbance in one's clock or circadian rhythm, a rhythm that your bowel needs to function properly.

Peristalsis is affected by time changes because it works on this circadian rhythm. The rising and setting of the sun affects the time at which your bowel contracts to move the contents out.

The healthier your bowel is, the less of a problem with this that you will have. The better formed your stools are, the less effort it takes to eliminate them. Water, fiber, and a familiar toilet are all helpful for elimination, but they are crutches that are not necessary when your bowel is healthy. If you suffer from persistent travelers constipation, it is a warning that your bowel is not as healthy as it could be.

Pregnancy and post-pregnancy constipation

This is a very common complaint and is mainly caused by physiological changes in the intestinal area and a resultant reduction in the strength of your bowel peristalsis. This is especially true after birth when "that whole area" has suffered stress, due to a difficult vaginal birth or C-section. An epidural and/ or the medications used during a C-section can also temporarily contribute to this problem.

High protein diets and constipation

High protein, low carbohydrate diets can be constipating because they reduce your body's cleansing process, which means they slow down the movement of acids, or trash, that enters your bowel. This was described earlier. This type of diet is likely responsible for the largest number of cases of prolonged constipation in this country, or going more than one day without having a bowel movement.

Bananas and constipation

Bananas are extremely easy to digest, alkalinizing, and abundant in beneficial minerals like potassium. Some people avoid eating them because they have heard they are constipating. Bananas help bind, or "soak up," acids in your bowel, so there are fewer free-floating acids that can trigger poorly formed stools. If you experience harder or less frequent stools when eating bananas, it is because prior to eating them, your stools were frequent and poorly formed. Frequent and poorly formed stools are worse than harder or less frequent ones. *Constipation is a good thing if you previously experienced loosely formed stools.* In other words, the consumption of the banana has improved, not worsened, your elimination.

Stop freaking out about constipation

I can't say this enough to clients who suffer from a history of constipation. Acids that have been formed into stools are not re-absorbed into your body, only the unformed acids are. When you are constipated it is not ideal, but it is significantly healthier than having frequent but poorly formed stools.

Chapter Seven

Healing Your Bowel

Healing your bowel entails rebuilding the bacterial environment within it. In this program, *Bowel Strength* and probiotics are used to accomplish this.

Your bowel will not simply heal itself.

Laxatives, colon cleansers, and other programs for the bowel do not heal it. When bowel-healing agents are used, an amount is utilized that is neither individualized nor strong enough to work.

Healing your bowel is a complex process that requires a great deal of information, knowledge and understanding. Also, the *correct* amount of the bowel-healing products needs to be taken in order for this to work. This chapter provides much of this information for you.

The necessity to actively heal your bowel

Exercise, colonics, fasting, eating more healthfully, diets, acupuncture, and 99% of the supplements and modalities that people use to look and feel better do not heal their bowel.

The April 12, 2006 edition of our local paper *The Daily Camera* highlighted the bacterial balance in the bowel. A local family nurse practitioner said that she understands the limited value of probiotics (i.e. using them after taking antibiotics), but that they shouldn't be taken all the time as "your really want to teach your body to make its own" and "it's best to try to do this through healthful eating." *That is utter nonsense.* I am certain this woman has never successfully helped someone heal his or her bowel.

If you throw rocks at your windows and they break, and then you stop throwing them, you will prevent *future* damage to your windows, but the damage that has already been done will not automatically fix itself. **The same holds true about your bowel. It will not fix itself; you must do something specifically for this to occur.** Only once your bowel has been healed can you depend on it to "make its own" beneficial bacteria. Maintaining bowel health and creating it are two entirely different situations. Maintaining a house and building one are also entirely different processes. **You must actively work to create bowel health.**

Bowel Strength and Probiotics Like Acidophilus Heal Your Bowel, *If Used Correctly*

I have spent thousands of hours over the last twenty years figuring out how to heal the bowel. I have seen thousands of clients and have worked on healing the bowel of every one of them. The information below is the result of my independent study and research. It is not documented anywhere else that I am aware of, although I would be more than happy to partake in such a process.

In my private practice the bacterial weakness in the bowel is taken care of with either one of two products—my product, *Bowel Strength*, or probiotics like acidophilus. (For sake of simplicity and due to its more recognizable name, when referring to probiotics I will often use the term acidophilus, even though this is only one of many strains of bacteria that can be classified as a probiotic). There may be other products that are helpful, but I specifically chose these two for their strength and convenience. Of the dozens of catalogues I receive from supplement manufacturers, *I have not found any product that works nearly as well as these.*

The benefits of *Bowel Strength* are as follows: It does not need to be refrigerated like acidophilus, making it more convenient. It is $25 to $30 a bottle less than a comparable amount of acidophilus. (I purchase it in very large quantities and pass my quantity discount on to you.) Finally, *Bowel Strength* contains some crutches that acidophilus does not, and clients appreciate having these to "hold them up" until their bowel is stronger.

The benefits of probiotics like acidophilus are as follows: It comes in capsule and powder form, whereas the *Bowel Strength* comes only in capsule form. For people who do not like to swallow pills, as well as for young children who can't, I recommend acidophilus. Depending on where you live, you may be able to find a strong, high quality brand at a local health food store, and this may be convenient for you. *Bowel Strength* needs to be ordered thorough me. For some, taking acidophilus is preferable, as it is a product they have heard of and for this reason, they may have more faith in it. Faith in healing your body is a necessity to succeed. With these clients I recommend acidophilus.

On the other hand, some clients have used acidophilus at a dose that was much to low to work, and this failure can be taken with them in the future as we work together and use the same product. For them, *Bowel Strength* is more effective. (Note: *Bowel Strength* contains black walnut hulls. While my experience and understanding is that these do not cause problems if one is allergic to walnuts, to be sure, use acidophilus instead, if you are.)

I purchase both of these products for clients and try to find the product that best serves their needs. I have many more clients who use *Bowel Strength* than acidophilus. If you don't know which one to take, don't worry. It is o.k. to try one and then switch to the other, either right away or later on in the process. What is most important right now is that you get in the car and start driving down the right road.

Fear of healing your bowel

It is extremely rare that I have a client for which these bowel-healing products do not suit their needs. When I have, the client has always presented themselves to me with a very unhealthy bowel and body, a long history of pain and discomfort, a past history of numerous failures at attempts to get better, and a crippling level of fear that caused them to distrust every product and every person who was trying to help them.

Fear and distrust are justified and understandable. But you cannot let it distract you from this process. If you are in this state, you must find some trust and strength to "try again." I am here today because I never gave up, even after dozens of failures to heal my body. You will never get down the road if you stop trying. That is a guarantee I can make to you.

How do *Bowel Strength* and acidophilus work? (it isn't what you think!)

Your bowel contains 100 trillion bacteria. Many of these are beneficial to the health of your body and are often referred to as the good bacteria. Acidophilus and bifidus are examples of good bacteria. Some of the bacteria in your bowel are harmful and are often referred to as bad bacteria. Yeast, Candida, and parasites are often lumped in with these bad bacteria. **To heal your bowel, it is important to create an environment that is conducive to the growth of the good bacteria, and discourages the growth of the bad bacteria.**

Bowel Strength

The most important ingredients in *Bowel Strength* are herbs that encourage the growth of these beneficial bacteria. These are herbs, like berberine and grapefruit seed extract, that affect the pH of your bowel and support the growth of healthy bacteria there. The healthy bacteria in your bowel will multiply if given some help. It's not as though they are all gone! Once they are plentiful enough, imagine that you have fixed the holes in your trashcan.

There are also a couple of ingredients in the *Bowel Strength* that treat your symptoms and do nothing to heal your bowel. For example, goldenseal acts like a natural antibiotic that helps kill off harmful germs, but it does not fix the weakness in your bowel that makes you vulnerable to bacterial infections in the first place. Gentian root is an anti-gas herb and wormwood and garlic, for example, help kill off bad bacteria as well. (A 1994 study showed that, in a test tube, garlic killed a variety of infectious organisms, including E. coli, streptococcus, and pneumonia.)

One of the most important bowel-healing ingredients in the *Bowel Strength* is berberine. This is a very strong herb and needs to be respected. You will find some warnings about it, and I couldn't agree more about them. I think that products containing it shouldn't be sold to the general public; an experienced health practitioner, like myself, who has used it with many clients and understands the benefits and risks, should be the only one dispensing it.

If you have any concerns about any of the ingredients in *Bowel Strength*, use acidophilus instead. I am not aware of any negative publicity concerning it. My belief is that the lack of negativity concerning it is not because it is better than a product with berberine, but because it is not nearly as strong, and it is simply marketed and researched much more aggressively. I prefer berberine because many of my clients present themselves to me with extremely unhealthy bowels, and if they do not use strong products, they fail to heal.

Acidophilus

Many people think that only probiotics like acidophilus can heal their bowel. They envision the good bacteria going into their bodies and setting up camp, but this is <u>not</u> how acidophilus works. *"Probiotics, such as L. acidophilus, produce lactic acid, which not only aids in digestion, but also creates an unfavorable environment for the proliferation of Candida albicans (yeast) and pathogenic bacteria in the digestive system. L. acidophilus also produces digestive enzymes that aid in the digestion, absorption, and assimilation of nutrients from food. This helps maintain a healthy intestinal tract, normalize bowel function, and decrease allergic reactions from food."*

(May 2006, *Naturopathic Doctor News & Review*).

Probiotics make your bowel less habitable for harmful bacteria by changing the chemistry of it. They also produce antimicrobial compounds that destroy pathogenic microbes. Killing off the bad guys leaves space for the good guys.

Acidophilus and *Bowel Strength* work the same way.

Like fertilizer for your lawn

Think of these products as fertilizer for your lawn. Some of the herbs in *Bowel Strength,* and probiotics like acidophilus, are fertilizer for your bowel bacteria. They help provide the ingredients needed for your good bacteria to multiply. A healthy lawn will keep weeds out, just as a healthy bowel will keep bad bacteria, Candida, parasites, and worms out.

They fix the holes in your roof

Bowel Strength and acidophilus "fix the holes in your roof." If you had no holes in your roof, your house would not get wet when it rained. If your bowel were strong, diet, stress, pollution, pesticides, etc, would not trigger symptoms and reactions. Every day that you take these products, envision workmen on your roof patching the holes. While all of these holes cannot be immediately fixed, over time, the cumulative effect of this action is that they all *will* be repaired.

How much should I take, and when?

If you are 18 years of age or older, start with 4 pills of *Bowel Strength* or 100 billion organisms of acidophilus/probiotics a day. The strength of probiotics is listed as a number of organisms per serving and can be found on the bottle. No one has, to my knowledge done a scientific comparison between these two products to determine how many *Bowel Strength* is equivalent, in strength, to acidophilus. From my own informal study, the amounts I have suggested are roughly equivalent, but this is not necessarily an accurate estimate.

If you take these products and your bowel movements remain relatively the same in three to four days, it is advisable that you increase the dosage. At this point try 8 pills/day of *Bowel Strength* or 250 billion organisms of probiotics a day. If this does not cause a change in your bowels in three to four days, try 12 *Bowel Strength* or 500 billion organisms of probiotics a day.

For children age 5-17, follow the above directions using one half (1/2) the suggested amounts. For advise for children under the age of 5, please contact me directly. I have helped many babies and toddlers, and most need help healing their bowel. In the future, look for *"This Works, Crutches Don't For Kids."*

You may not be tolerating these products/they may be too strong, and therefore not needed, if the following occurs one to two days after introducing them or increasing the dosage: your bowel movements become more frequent, you become more gassy, and/or your stools become mushier and/or looser.

These reactions do not guarantee that they are too strong and unneeded, but imply it is a possibility, and if this happens to you, you must explore this possibility. Taking these products when you don't need them and/or if they are too strong will make you look and feel worse, not better.

If your stools tend to be loose before you begin the program, it is much harder to determine when the supplements are too strong. One clue can be the frequency of elimination. If your bowel movements become more frequent, it is also possible that the supplements are too strong.

If you react to these supplements as described above within one to two days of starting them, stop them altogether and try the same dose again in four to five days. Loose bowels will occur if your bowel bacteria are strong and these items are not needed, but loose bowels can occur for many other reasons as well. The same holds true for increased gas. If you start the pills at the same time that you increase your fiber intake, fruit intake, or reduce your protein intake, these items, and not the *Bowel Strength* or acidophilus, could cause gas. If your stools become firmer off the pills but then become loose again when you re-try the dosage, it is likely that it is the pills that are too strong.

Because it is very important to find the dosage that is right for you, and it is very important that you "blame the right thing" when you start these products, do not change your diet at all for the first three days. Likewise, try not to introduce or increase these at a time when your stress levels are noticeably different. Do not start this program right before a move, or a vacation. If you lost your cat and can't sleep, don't start them then either, for example.

At the start of this program, it is rare for a new client to find that 12 Bowel Strength or 500 billion organisms of acidophilus a day, is too strong.

I have worked with many clients who have taken over 24 pills /day of *Bowel Strength* or over 800 billion organisms of acidophilus/day without it becoming too strong. These amounts have proven to be remarkably healing. Even still, many of these clients have needed to take this dosage for one or two years to really noticeably heal their bowel and body. If these same clients had taken only 4 pills/day of *Bowel Strength*, it would have taken six times longer to see results, or six to twelve years. This is why it is incredibly important to take a dose that is strong enough. Not many people will have the dedication or patience to stay with a program for six or twelve years, and most importantly, there is a safe way to heal much faster than this.

The more of these products that you tolerate, the less healthy your bowel is. The more there is to fix, the more complicated this becomes.

If you tolerate 12 pills of *Bowel Strength* a day or 500 billion organisms of acidophilus, and you want to go faster, I advise you to seek help along this journey. You can contact me at donna@ThisWorksCrutchesDont.com.

All of the supplements I recommend—*Bowel Strength*, acidophilus and the crutches listed in Chapter 10—are in doses higher than the standard recommendations. In my experience this is not only safe, but also a necessity, temporarily, to get results. For more information on using high dosages of these products, please refer to Chapter 10.

Going too slowly?

When you go too slowly and take a much smaller amount of these supplements than you need, you will be uncomfortable, unhealthy, symptomatic, and overweight longer than necessary due to your unhealthy bowel. You will have to live in your crumbling, out-dated house longer than you need to. You are also traveling at a speed that will take you a long time to get maximum results, including weight loss. Finally, the weakness of your bowel bacteria leaves you vulnerable to illness and other discomforts.

Going too fast?

When you go too fast, you are uncomfortable as well. If you try to drive towards your destination at 200 mph, you are likely to crash, miss your exit, or get thrown into jail for excessive speeding; in other words, you are unlikely to reach your destination faster than if you go slower. If you take too many of these supplements, and do not follow my instructions, you are more likely to fail as well.

The best amount of these supplements to use is that elusive "100 mph" one, the amount that produces bowel healing as fast as is comfortably possible.

Unfortunately, many variables affect this dosage and it is unrealistic to expect to be able to maintain this ideal amount steadily throughout this program.

Going too fast is uncomfortable, but going too slowly is uncomfortable, too. Most of my clients drive too slowly.

Going too fast is much more common later into this program.

Loose stools and diarrhea: is this from the products or something else?

Every year, over 75 million people become ill from eating contaminated food. One of the most common symptoms of food poisoning is diarrhea occurring more than twice a day. When you have diarrhea you lose a lot of valuable water and electrolytes, which can lead to dehydration, even death. Diarrhea is a symptom that a strong toxin is in your bowel, and your body is sending water into it in an attempt to dilute it.

Given the large numbers of reported illness caused by food poisoning every year, it is very likely that one of you will be subject to a food-borne pathogen in the near future. If this happens before you have healed your bowel, you will need help. If you experience loose, watery stools more than 2x/day for more than two days in a row, and you have stopped the *Bowel Strength* or acidophilus, you might have food poisoning. A trip to your doctor is imperative if diarrhea continues more than two days in a row. Healing will not yield persistent diarrhea, so never assume that this is the problem.

The flu virus can also trigger loose stools. If your stools are loose and you have a fever, it is almost always due to the flu and not due to the products you are taking. Bacterial infections can produce loose stools, too, and if you have travelled out of the country—to Mexico, Peru, China, Chile, India, etc ---and your stools have become loose, it is very likely that you picked up an infection or parasite while travelling.

More loose stool triggers

Blaming *Bowel Strength* or acidophilus for every case of loose stools will at best cause you to heal much too slowly; at worst, it can lead you to wrongly attribute the condition to these products and stop the healing process altogether.

If your stools become loose, it may be that you have holes in your roof and it is raining hard. If may be that there is too much acidity in your weak bowel. While the bowel-healing products will cause loose stools when they are too strong, the majority of the time that a client has loose stools, it is being triggered by another variable.

If your stools are loose, avoid the following for the next few days and see if these are causing the problem: stress, fruit, spicy foods, beans, chocolate, dairy products (especially milk and ice cream), coffee, alcohol, sugar, and red meat.

The item on this list that most of my clients seem to disregard is the high consumption of fruit. Fruit is "good for you," so how could it cause loose stools? This is a common question. Fruit *is* good for you, but fruit is very cleansing. It causes a lot of acidity to be "sent into" your bowel. This is good for the other organs of your body, because the more acids that are in your bowel, the fewer that are stored in your organs, causing damage and disease. Nevertheless, many people do not have a strong bowel, and throwing too much acidity into it by eating a lot of fruit triggers loose stools.

In the summertime, when fruit is especially plentiful, I run into this scenario often. The fruits that seem most likely to trigger loose stools are cherries, oranges and nectarines, peaches, berries, pineapple, dried fruit, plums, apricots, and mangos, however this is not an exclusive listing. If your stools are loose, try eating no fruit except bananas, for a couple days and see if that changes things. If it does, it will prevent you from wrongly blaming the *Bowel Strength* or acidophilus, and this is very important. **Wrongly blaming the products for causing loose stools is a common reason for failing to heal your body.**

In summary, if you have holes in your trashcan and you throw trash into it, it will leak out over the ground. If your bowel bacteria are weak, eating cleansing foods like fruit, high fiber, and high carbohydrate foods, can cause more acids to enter it than it can handle, and this results in loose stools.

Diarrhea is a possible side effect of a number of medications, too. If you have recently started a new one and your stools become loose, check with your doctor to see if this is a possible side-effect and if so, find out if there is another medication that you can take that won't cause this to happen.

An increase in stress can also trigger loose stools if your bowel is unhealthy. This can be a hard variable to control, in which case, if you stop the supplements and your stools continue to be too loose, think about what is happening in your life. Is a relative ill, have you been worried about your job, did you lose a lot of money in the stock market, has your dog run away, or have any other unusually stressful conditions been going on?

If you have frequent, loose stools the following supplements also need to be avoided: vitamin C, aloe, senna, mineral oil, cascara sagrada, rhubarb, and magnesium. If you take a calcium supplement if may also contain magnesium. Check the label for the main ingredients and if magnesium is included, stop the supplement for a few days and see if your bowels are less frequent and/or better formed off of it. Remember, it is better to have only one bowel movement a day than two if they are loose. If your stools are better, and you still want to take calcium, get a calcium supplement without additional magnesium. If your stools are not better off the magnesium then it is ok to add it back.

Recently a multi-level marketing company has been selling a product that contains aloe. The other day a client who suffers from loose stools and hemorrhoids found out for herself that aloe should be avoided. A friend sold her this product and, not surprisingly, it aggravated her hemorrhoids.

For more information on the necessity of avoiding vitamin C when your stools are loose, see Chapter 10.

Respect these products

It is very important to respect these products when they are too strong. Do not perceive this as negative; the truth is, it is very positive. When these are too strong, it is your body's way of saying they are not needed. Taking something your body does not need will slow down the healing, not speed it up.

Taking too many of these supplements can be harmful if done for a period of time. And while I have had pregnant women do this program, it has always been under my careful guidance and it has proved beneficial, not harmful. If you are trying this on your own, do not use these products if you are pregnant.

Ultimately, the quantity of supplements that you take has nothing to do with how quickly you proceed through this program. Often I see clients who get confused by this concept and many who believe that more is always better. This is not true. Thinking that you can take a stronger dosage that causes diarrhea and get through this program faster is foolish. You will not succeed if you are impatient and attempt this. Trying to force your body to heal at a pace that is faster than it can handle is very disrespectful to your body and needs to be completely avoided.

Rather than becoming impatient with the process, be grateful that there is an answer. Be grateful that your ill health and weight problems are not permanent conditions that cannot be changed. I completely destroyed my health when I was growing up and healing it gave me another life. I am grateful that there was a way to reverse all of my mistakes. Be grateful that you can completely change the health of your body as well, and know that everyday you follow this program you are healing and making permanent, cumulative changes towards health; you are not just treating your symptoms with crutches and feeling better, but actually becoming less healthy.

On the other hand, don't worry about using these products. Millions of people have died who were not using them! In other words, it is much safer to try to heal your body than to not try at all.

Taking the correct amount of these products is a necessity for success

The specific brand of acidophilus is not nearly as important as taking the right amount and using it correctly. **The correct application of a product is what makes it work.** People who have used other products to heal their bowel and failed have done so because of the way they were using the product, not because the product was ineffective.

As I like to say, Van Gogh could use the cheapest paints around and still paint a much more spectacular picture than most of us, even if we were using the highest quality paints available.

A number of books and health practitioners claim to heal your bowel, but this is not true. Just because you advise someone to take probiotics does not mean that you have healed your bowel. The correct amount of probiotics, or *Bowel Strength*, is a necessity to achieve this, and so far, I have never seen a recommendation made that does this.

If you want to retire in ten years you must save money. But the amount you save every month is paramount to you achieving this goal. Simply saving money is not enough. If you make $5000 a month and save $1 a month, you will never be able to retire in ten years. You have saved too little and will not be able to meet your goal. If you save $5000 every month, you will also fail, as you won't have enough money every month to buy food and pay your bills and you will starve and die! Again, "saving money" did not allow you to reach your goal.

If you want to heal your bowel you must take a probiotic or *Bowel Strength*, but this alone is not enough to accomplish this either. *If you take too few or too many probiotics or Bowel Strength, you will fail to heal your bowel and body.*

When you heal, one size does not fit all: your needs are unique

Any book or individual that recommends a "one size fits all" approach to acidophilus is not qualified to advise you on how to heal your bowel. When you treat symptoms with crutches, you can safely give everyone the same amount of a supplement. You are used to this approach. It cannot be used when you heal.

I can see fifty people with the exact same symptoms who need completely different amounts of *Bowel Strength and* acidophilus, as well as time, to heal. Yet over and over again, I see recommendations made for these products based on symptoms rather than individuals. For example, everyone with Irritable Bowel Syndrome will be told to take the same amount for the same time period. "Follow the directions on the bottle (of probiotics)," writes a naturopath in a nutrition journal. These approaches simply don't work, at least not for the vast majority of people who follow them.

If you throw a handful of mud at the wall some will stick and much will fall off. If you tell everyone with a certain symptom to take the same thing it will work for some, but for many more, it won't. Sadly, many of these people will then conclude that there is no hope for them.

When I was sick I was always the mud that fell off. I always heard that I was the difficult case that didn't respond like everyone else. Knowing what I do now I understand that the biggest problem was the program I was on, but there definitely was a degree of failure due to the lack of knowledge of the professional in applying the information on an individual basis.

Also, do not compare yourself to your friends or family who have gone through or are going through this program, and never assume you need the same amount that they are taking.

You won't know if you need them until you try them

It is important to try *Bowel Strength* or acidophilus even if you think your bowel is healthy. *One to two days after trying these, your stools will <u>not</u>*

become loose or more frequent if your bowel is unhealthy and you need to heal it. (As little as one billion organisms of acidophilus or one capsule of *Bowel Strength* per day will produce loose stools and discomfort in an individual with a healthy bacterial environment.)

It is a lack of an immediate bowel reaction to the supplements that means you need them! It means these products are needed, and if you keep taking them, your bowel and body will heal and become healthier. *It means that if you do not take them, your struggles with your weight, health, addictions, and illness will be much greater than is necessary.*

We are used to taking pills and immediately responding, because they are crutches that treat symptoms, so this concept can be very different and confusing. However, it is an extremely important one to follow in order for this process to work.

Remember, an unhealthy bowel may produce somewhat normal bowel movements which can lead you to believe that your bowel is healthy and this program cannot help you, or is not needed, but don't be fooled. If your trashcan has a thousand holes in it but you never throw trash into it, you may think that your trashcan is in good shape, too! I have worked with a number of clients who have come in with cancer, autoimmune diseases; weight problems, etc, who thought their bowel was healthy because their elimination wasn't too bad. Once we started the *Bowel Strength* however, they found they could take a large amount without getting a reaction. This is a true measure of the health of your bowel.

If you haven't taken this much acidophilus in the past, or have used a product similar to the *Bowel Strength* at a lower dosage for a short period of time, do not discount their ability to help you. I have a client who used a similar product for only one month, at 9/day. For over ten years, she struggled to get well. When she came to me she still had a very weak immune system—brain fog, dizziness, fatigue—and she responded very well to a dosage of 14/day for twenty months. She is a completely new woman.

When do I take these products?

While some product labels and practitioners recommend that these products be taken with meals, my clients get the best results when they are taken on an empty stomach. For this purpose, an empty stomach is defined as ten or more minutes before a meal or thirty or more minutes after a meal. If you forget a dose or cannot follow these guidelines, it is much better to take them with meals than to not take them at all.

The total amount that you take in a day should be divided into two dosages. These times do not need to be exactly twelve hours apart. Simply aim for half of the dose in the morning and the other half in the late afternoon or evening. It is not important to keep these times consistent from one day to the next. And if you would like to take these products more often that is great, although not necessary. For example, you could split your 9/day dosage into three doses of three pills each time.

How to Obtain *Bowel Strength* and Probiotics

Bowel Strength is my private label product and can be ordered online through www.ThisWorksCrutchesDont.com. Please see this site for pricing and shipping information. There is also an order form for it at the end of this book.

Probiotics, like acidophilus, can be found in health food stores. They are usually in a small refrigerator in the supplement section of the store. The disadvantage of purchasing acidophilus at the health food store is that currently, the majority of them do not carry products that are very strong. The low strength means that you will need to take *a lot* of pills every day for them to do you much good. You can also purchase probiotics from the company I use. These are hypoallergenic, very high quality, and very strong. Their strength means you take fewer pills. Their cost is usually less than a comparable strength from a health food store. **"Ther-Biotic Complete Powder"** (product code K-TCP) is powdered and contains 100 billion organisms of probiotics per ¼ teaspoon. **"Ther-Biotic Detoxification Support"** (product code V770-06) comes in capsule form and contains 50 billion organisms per pill. To order these products, call **Prothera at 1-775-850-8800. You will need authorization code #276** to place this order. These products arrive cold and need to be refrigerated upon receipt, like all probiotics.

The application of the product matters a lot more than the product itself

I have found that many different brands of acidophilus work *if used correctly, at the correct dosage*. This is significantly more important than the product that is used. When I see a client who has used or is still using acidophilus, it has always been at a dosage that is completely insufficient to quickly heal their bowel and body. Sadly, this had led many to believe that these products cannot heal.

If you ever see a health practitioner or read a book or article in which it is claimed that there is only "one magic product" to achieve a health benefit, run away! This is not true.

Over the years I have seen many companies market their acidophilus product as the "one that will work because it contains some special formulation," but in my experience, this is simply a marketing tool to get you to purchase their product. I have had clients use many different products from many different companies over the years and they all work well. *The key to getting results from acidophilus is using it correctly, not using one particular brand versus another.* There are many different brands of saws that will cut your tree down for you; but a saw sitting around in your garage won't cut your tree for you. You need to get it out and use it correctly in order to achieve your goal.

Also, many acidophilus products contain a strain of several more beneficial bacteria—like L. bifidus, L.rhamnosus, L. casei, B. breve, S. thermophilus, and B. lactis. These are all good products, but including numerous strains of bacteria do not necessarily make these better products than ones that contain only one or two. The total number of organisms per capsule of *all* the strains of bacteria combined should be counted when determining how much to use. If a product contains five different strains of beneficial bacterial and each one provides 1 billion organisms per capsule, then each capsule contains a total of 5 billion bacteria. In other words, do not only count the acidophilus when determining the strength. A few acidophilus products also contain a small amount of other ingredients, like ginger, FOS, barley greens, and citrus pectin. All of these are fine, but are not to be counted towards the strength of the product. They are listed as milligrams per serving versus organisms per serving.

If your bowel is very weak you may be sensitive to acidophilus products that contain wheat and/or dairy. If you get gassy or cramps after using acidophilus, you may be sensitive to that product. It does not necessarily mean you do not need it, on the contrary. If your bowel were stronger you would not react to wheat and dairy. If this happens to you, consider ordering the acidophilus that I listed earlier. It is allergen free and my most sensitive clients tolerate it well.

I am leery of probiotics that do not need to be refrigerated after opening, and I suggest you stay away from these, as their strength is questionable.

What to Expect as You Heal Your Bowel

Form improves before frequency

As your bowel health improves, the form will continuously improve as well. The frequency, however, will first slow down, that is, if you start off with frequent but poorly formed stools. Your bowel movements may become slower or your stools may become harder, *temporarily*. Temporary constipation due to healing your bowel is a positive reaction that is often perceived as negative. When you heal, your bowel movements will not slow down significantly. You will not go only once every three days or more, for example. To understand why this happens and why it is beneficial, go back to that description of the how stools are formed in Chapter 6. A very unhealthy bowel produces loose, frequent stools. A healthier bowel produces firmer, less frequent ones. The healthiest bowel produces frequent, well-formed stools. If you start off in California with a very unhealthy bowel, you will have to drive through Kansas and a healthier bowel, to get to Massachusetts and the healthiest bowel. You cannot avoid it.

It is much healthier, and you are eliminating more acidity, if you go every other day and your stool is wide and hard then if you go every day and your stools are skinny or too short. I get phone calls from clients frequently when they reach this stage, even though I have explained beforehand that it will occur, that it is positive, and it won't last forever. When this happens, clients look and feel better than they did before. The infrequent elimination, however, seems to evoke a state of fear and mental discomfort. Ironically, the true fear should occur when there are frequent but poorly formed stools. This is the most dangerous elimination, but for some reason, we have not been conditioned to be fearful of it. When you reach this stage, as long as you continue with healing your bowel, you will move out of it and toward a much healthier elimination. Keep driving the car, and eventually you will get to the ideal elimination.

If you reach this state it is confirmation that you need the *Bowel Strength* or acidophilus, it is not too strong, and if you keep taking it, your bowel and body will heal and become healthier.

However, if you are new to this program—you have done it for less than six months and/or this change in your bowel movements occurs with other new symptoms, like rectal bleeding, fever, or pain—it is possible that your bowel was very weak when you began this process and that this new bowel scenario is a reflection of this weakness; it could be something serious that needs medial attention. In all of the years that I have done his work this has never happened to one of my clients, but it is much easier to make this assessment individually than it is through a book, of course. The only incident that I can recall is once when a new client came to me with a very unhealthy bowel and a few days later, *before we had even started the program,* he had severe intestinal discomfort and diarrhea that required medical intervention. It was discovered at that time that he had some serious health issues. Once he got over this crisis he came back in and has been doing very well and has not had a repeat of his original problem since.

These above concepts can be very confusing and unexpected when they occur. For this reason, it would be advisable that you re-read this section if this situation does happen.

Less symptoms and weight but a temporary worsening of your bowel movements

Once your bowel has become stronger and your symptoms change and improve, you may also experience a temporary worsening of your bowel movements. As you become healthier there will be an increased movement of acids into your bowel, and the true health of it may be exposed. Once the trash from your organs began moving into your bowel, you may discover that it wasn't as great as you thought! This usually manifests as increased sensitivity to highly acidic foods like alcohol, sugar, or coffee. This happens even though you may not have had this reaction, of loose stools, after consuming these foods before starting this program. It is important to stop these foods for a few days to see if they are causing your loose stools before you blame the *Bowel Strength* or probiotics.

You are healing your bowel even if your bowel movements do not immediately improve

It can be very difficult to take these products when you do not immediately respond positively to them. This is one of the hardest parts of this program, this lack of instant gratification. You have to keep buying and swallowing something even though you cannot immediately see the benefit of doing so. The lack of immediate response to this product does not mean it is not working. It works. It just means your bowel is unhealthy.

You need to have discipline and consider the long-term benefits. If you want to retire in ten years you have to have the discipline to save money every month so this can happen. Every month you have to put money aside—money that could have otherwise been spent on toys and vacations—so that when you retire you don't have to continue working; so that you can enjoy it. You have to view the *Bowel Strength* and acidophilus the same way. Your discipline in taking them daily allows you to reach a time when you can effortlessly look and feel great and be free of disease.

Cumulatively, and gradually, you *will* experience the benefits of these products. If you have 10,000 holes in your roof and fix ten of these you won't notice this; once 1,000 are fixed, you will. Only after you have made significant progress in healing your bowel will you notice that your bowel movements have improved.

See Chapter 8 for information on taking bentonite, a product you should take while you are healing your bowel and body as it can immediately improve the form and frequency of your bowel movements and as a result, greatly expedite the elimination of acids from your body as you heal your bowel.

The workmen still work when it's raining

As you are healing your bowel, envision many workmen on the roof repairing the holes that are in it. It will take some time to repair all of them, and inevitably, there will be times when a lot of rain hits your roof. For example, you have friends in town and eat more and drink more than usual. When this rain hits your roof, your house will get wet; symptoms may flare-up. This does not mean that your roof is weaker or that the *Bowel Strength or* acidophilus are not working. **The appearance of a symptom does not mean that healing is not happening. It means you have not completed the healing process, so keep going!**

Longer breaks are fine; just get back in the car eventually

If you need to stop these supplements for more than one week, for whatever reason, that is fine. You can start and stop the process anytime you want. You will not go backwards if you do. You will simply pick right back up from where you left off. If you drive your car for 1,000 miles and stop, your car does not roll backwards! When you are ready to drive again you will be starting at the 1,000-mile mark.

If you stop the supplements it is perfectly ok to re-start them at the same dosage that you were taking when you stopped. You will not need to work your way up to it like you did initially. Some clients stop these supplements when they are traveling so that they don't have to bother with them. I always encourage that.

Most importantly, when you do stop, make sure that you get back in the car and keep driving towards your destination of ideal health and weight. **Taking a break if needed is great as long as you come back and finish the job. Do not view these breaks as a failure, and know that you can always "come back and finish up where you let off."**

Just keep driving!

If *Bowel Strength* or a powerful acidophilus become too expensive or difficult for you to take aggressively, simply take less and go slower. While this path takes longer, compared to the wrong path that most people are on—traveling 25 mph in the *wrong* direction—even if you only drive 25 mph in the *right* direction, you are in a great place; you are making great progress towards your ideal health and weight. *This is not an all or nothing program. Your bowel will not heal by itself. If you tolerate these products, you need to take them.*

The End of the Road: The Need to Decrease and Eventually Stop These Products

Every application of these products that I have seen has wrongly focused on using them as crutches versus supplements to heal your bowel and body. The standard recommended amounts are completely insufficient to quickly heal the average person's bowel. If someone needs to take 500 billion organisms of probiotics a day for two years to heal their bowel and they take only the standard amount of 5 billion a day, it *would* take "forever" to heal at this amount.

These supplements are strong but inappropriate to take long-term. When used as I suggest, they will need to be stopped at some point. They are harmful to take long-term. I have never had someone do this, at least not while I was working with them, so I cannot say for sure what the consequence would be, but I feel certain it would be harmful. Will this happen? Most likely it won't or can't happen. When they become too strong, you will be too uncomfortable to continue with them.

As your bowel becomes healthier you need to reduce these products

Once you have found an amount of *Bowel Strength* or probiotics that you need and tolerate, you cannot simply take that amount indefinitely. You have to pay attention to your bowels and body *throughout this program*. As your bowel becomes healthier it will need, and tolerate, smaller amounts of these products. If you have taken 12 *Bowel Strength* a day for 11 months and your stools become loose, you need to consider that this dosage might need to be reduced. Try half this amount, or 6/day, for five days or so and see if your bowels improve. If so, perhaps it is time to reduce your dosage. To be sure, a week later, re-try the higher amount and see if this triggers loose stools in one or two days. If so, it is time to reduce your dosage. If not, it is not time to reduce your dosage. Follow the same instructions for the probiotics, cutting them in half if your stools become loose, and re-testing this a week later. The healthier your bowel is, the fewer of these products you will be able to take, and the fewer you will need to "drive 100 mph."

You will definitely need to reduce these as your bowel becomes healthier, but it is unlikely to happen within the first six months of taking them. Follow the instructions given earlier for loose stools if this occurs to you and you have used these products for fewer than six months.

Kick the workmen out for a while: stop these products for one week every two months

Stop the supplements for one week every two months to confirm that the amount you are currently taking is not too strong. While loose stools are a sign that they are too strong, it is *not* always that obvious. The supplements can get a little too strong and create some discomforts, but not be strong enough to produce loose stools.

When you use a crutch, like most other supplements, you will feel worse when you stop it. If your leg is broken and you use crutches to get around and the next day you decide not to use them, you will not be able to get around. Most of you have had this experience because the vast majority of you are using crutches now.

Bowel Strength and acidophilus are *not* crutches. They heal. If you remodel half of your house and then kick out the workmen, the half that was remodeled will stay remodeled. It doesn't just fall apart because the workmen leave. **You won't feel worse if you stop; you can only feel the same or better.**

Here is a comment I hear often: "I was taking eight *Bowel Strength* a day and my bowels were doing great and I was feeling great. I stopped the product and a few weeks later my stools got worse again. Does this mean I will need this product forever to keep my bowels good?" If your stools become worse when you stop the *Bowel Strength* or acidophilus, it is not because you will need these products forever. You won't. If your stools become worse when you stop it has no direct correlation to stopping; it is simply a coincidence in timing. It means you have not yet finished healing your bowel.

When you stop the supplements you are looking for a positive change in your bowels after a few days. Are your stools slower or harder? Are you less gassy? Do you feel better? If yes, then perhaps the amount you were on was getting to be too much. If you get this reaction, re-try the amount you were on prior to stopping and see if you feel worse in two days. If you do, it is even more likely that the supplement was getting too strong. In this case, reduce the supplement to a dosage that is 50% of your previous one and stay there until that also becomes too strong.

If you re-try the previous higher dosage and you do not feel uncomfortable with it after a couple days, you obviously don't want to attribute your improvements off of it to the fact that it was too strong, so go back to your original amount. If you feel exactly the same off of them, and if your bowels are exactly the same as well, then after the week is up, go back to the same dosage that you were on when you stopped.

An added benefit of stopping these supplements every once in a while is so that you can experience the permanence of the healing that you have created. It allows you to truly grasp what I am saying. For some of my clients it is when they stop and find that the improvements they achieved on them remain, that they finally get the difference between this program of healing and other programs that only treat symptoms with crutches.

Sometimes you go faster when you go slower. Do not view these breaks as non-productive. They allow you to make sure you are on the right road. Once you are certain of this, you can speed up with confidence. **Impatience is the hardest disease to cure. Don't let it lead you to failure.**

What does the finish line look like?

Do not stop these products just because your symptoms, weight, or bowels are doing well. **Stop when 4 *Bowel Strength* a day or 50 billion organisms of acidophilus a day causes your stools to become loose. In other words, stop them when they are no longer needed; not when you feel or look better. You may look or feel better and still have weakness in your bowel or body.**

It is complicated but worth it

I can guarantee there will be a number of times during this process that you become confused and frustrated. You will get lost on the road many times. If there was a simple answer to our health and weight problems we would all be healthy and at our ideal weight. The answer exists. It will take patience and persistence for you to achieve it. The end of this road is far better than you can imagine and worth fighting for.

If you have gotten lost, contact me at www.ThisWorksCrutchesDont.com to schedule an appointment.

How Long Will it Take to Heal My Bowel, and How Long Will it Remain Healed?

You have 10 trillion cells in your body and 100 trillion bacteria in your bowel. That is 100,000,000,000. This is a very large, inconceivable number. What if only 1/10 of your bowel bacteria are unhealthy? How long would it take to "fix" 10 trillion bacteria? It would take a while.

It takes time to heal your bowel and body, but it takes a lot to weaken it. You can heal your bowel and body much faster than the time it took for it to become unhealthy. If your bowel has been unhealthy for forty years and it takes two to heal it, this is a lot faster than forty years. If you have been sick for ten years you can't reverse that in ten days. People will promise you that it can be done, but it cannot. You will find that out for yourself if you fall for these promises.

On a daily basis, when your bowel movements do not meet the ideal description given in Chapter 6, some acids are not eliminated and are instead stored in your body. How many days, weeks, and years has this occurred for you? In a very short time, you are trying to get out all of the acids that have taken decades to build up in your body.

If you inherited an unhealthy intestinal bacterial environment as a baby (and most likely you did), and you have a lot of holes in your trashcan, it will take some time to fix this.

The time and money you spend on this program is limited and will be significantly less than the time and money you will spend, and have already spent, on crutches.

The length of time it takes to heal your bowel is variable from one individual to the next. For some, this occurs in six months, and for others, it will take two years or longer. The variables listed below describe some of the circumstances that affect the length of the program.

Are you focused on one symptom or do you want to eliminate all of them?

Do you want to remodel your kitchen only, even though the rest of the house needs help too, or do you want to do the whole house? The kitchen alone will take less time than remodeling the entire house.

Most clients don't come in with the goal of completely healing their bowel and body, because they don't know that this is possible, and they don't know how healthy they can be. If a client has high cholesterol, for example, and that resolves itself, she may not realize that her allergies can be eliminated as well. For her, success may be defined as the lowering of her cholesterol, and achieving this may take only six months. She may "stop" the process once this is achieved and not completely heal her body and eliminate the allergies. So the length of this program is affected by your ultimate goal. Are you interested in eliminating one symptom, or do you want to completely heal your body and eliminate all them? If you choose the later, it will take longer to accomplish this.

I had a client who came to me about four years ago because she suffered from frequent diarrhea. She spent about six months healing her bowel so it was strong enough for the diarrhea to stop, but then she stopped the program. She came back recently and the diarrhea was still gone, but the weaknesses that she never finished healing still existed. She still had yeast infections, for example. In other words, her initial objective took only six months to correct; but this did not mean her bowel and body had been entirely healed. This takes longer.

The weakness of your bowel to start with

Most babies come into the world with unhealthy bowels. I have worked with a number of young infants in this situation. They have not lived long enough to "damage their bowels" by stress or diet. Their poor elimination is purely inherited. Most of you probably inherited unhealthy bowels too.

How long has it been since you've had consistently well-formed stools? The longer it has been, the longer it will take to heal your bowel. Luckily, if you are 50 years old and have never had healthy bowel movements, it will take a lot less time than 50 years to heal it.

How much of the *Bowel Strength* or acidophilus you tolerate

The more you can tolerate, the weaker your bowel, and the longer it will take to heal. I know this seems backwards. Most people would expect that the more they take the faster it would go, but it doesn't work that way with healing your bowel. The more you can tolerate, the less healthy your bowel is, and the longer it takes to heal it. The more you can tolerate, the longer the road that you need to travel. Because there are only 24 hours in a day and you can only drive so fast, it will take some time to get down it.

Your symptoms

Do you have a history of dairy or other food allergies or intolerances? If yes, your bowel is very unhealthy and it will take some time to fix. Do you experience hemorrhoids or diarrhea more than twice a month? Your bowel is very unhealthy. Diverticulitis, a history of colon cancer, Colitis, Chron's disease, polyps—these all happen when your bowel is very unhealthy and will take some time to heal.

In most cases, symptoms of a very unhealthy body correspond to a very unhealthy bowel as well. Arthritis, clogged arteries, autoimmune diseases, osteoporosis, diabetes, migraines, cancer, liver disease, high blood pressure, and all chronic and fatal illnesses are going to take a lot longer to eliminate than conditions like acne, frequent colds, gas, and headaches, which are conditions associated with a relatively healthier body.

If you have weight or health symptoms even though you are using crutches, be very patient!

When I see a new client with health or weight complaints and they are already heavily using a "crutch," I know I'm in for a tough time with this person. These situations indicate that their underlying system is extremely unhealthy to begin with. If someone has migraines and is eating a high protein diet, the high protein diet "crutch" isn't working too well, which means their bowel is extremely unhealthy. If someone comes to me and is taking numerous supplement crutches and they are ill or overweight, again, I know that their bowel is very unhealthy and we have a lot of work to do.

If two clients come to see me with the same symptoms, like eczema, but one eats a high protein diet or takes a lot of supplements, and the other eats a low protein diet or takes no supplements, the later person will see results much faster. The later person has a much healthier system to begin with.

If you have tried a lot of supplements, reduce your carbohydrate intake, minimize wheat or dairy, and/or drink a lot of water, and you still have symptoms, you are in bad shape. When commercials say, "When diet and exercise are not enough, you need to take medication," they are, in part, referring specifically to people with very weak bowels for whom the crutches aren't working.

If the crutch isn't working, the underlying problem is quite bad and it will take a while to fix. If either of these conditions applies to you, you will need to be very patient with this process. As always, however, I would urge you to be grateful there is an answer, because without one, you would be at high risk of a deadly or debilitating illness.

Or need to exercise frequently to keep your weight off

Likewise, a healthy body will maintain a healthy weight without the need for exercise to "do that for you." The more dependent you are on the exercise crutch for weight loss or symptoms reduction, the weaker your bowel is and the longer this process will take. If you need to exercise more than thirty minutes a day more than twice a week, your bowel is unhealthy. If you need to exercise one hour four or more times a week to maintain your weight, your bowel is even less healthy. If you stop exercising and gain three to five pounds in one month, your bowel is unhealthy. If you stop exercising and gain more than five pounds or more in a month, it is even less healthy and it will take longer to heal it. You are also at high risk if you don't.

The weakness of your other organs

The greater the accumulation of acidity in your body, the longer it will take to heal your bowel. This acidity will be sent into your bowel to be eliminated as you heal your bowel and body, and this will cause continued stress to your bowel. If there is a lot of trash in your house, it will need to be emptied out through your trashcan. Your trashcan, or bowel, will be "working hard" to support this.

Your bowel is a gigantic organ/trashcan and it is necessary to support it through the healing process because it is not designed to handle "so much trash at one time." Your trash has slowly been accumulating and you are trying to eliminate it very quickly, relatively speaking. You are starting this program with less than ideal bowel health, and so it is absolutely normal and natural for you to have to spend many months "helping" your bowel.

How long you have had other symptoms, including struggles with your weight

If you are trying to eliminate a condition that has occurred only in the last two months, you will generally see this go away much faster than if you are trying to eliminate something that you have struggled with for the last twenty years.

How fast you go

My goal is to help my clients drive down the healing road at "100 mph." This is my analogy for healing at a pace that is neither too slow nor too fast. There are several reasons a client will fail to do this: One, it is not important to them to heal as quick as possible; two, they are fearful of the healing process and tend to go too slow because of it; three, they cannot afford to go as fast as possible or choose not to make healing their body a financial priority; and four, some clients have such a weakness in their bowel that going 100 mph is not possible. They reach the maximum number of *Bowel Strength* or acidophilus that I allow before it gets too strong. If you are one of these people and would like to go faster, contact me at www.ThisWorksCrutchesDont. com and I can work with you individually to accomplish this. The more pills you take, the more important it is that you do so under the guidance of someone who can safely direct you down this road. I have yet to meet another practitioner who has this experience, but perhaps there are others out there. If you are one and are reading this, please let me know so that I may share your name with others.

How many breaks you take

I advise you to take a break from the bowel supplements every two months. For some, these breaks will be more frequent—forgetting to take the pills, reducing them too quickly out of fear, running out of them, discontinuing them because of a family, personal, financial or other crisis—all of these can occur and add time to the length of the program. Very few of my clients "drive down the healing road at 100 mph" the entire time. It is much more difficult to do this than you may think. Likewise, many of my clients have dramatically changed their lives with this program, so taking breaks is by no means a deterrent to the effectiveness of this.

Give it time

The vicious cycle of health and healing is one people are especially vulnerable to when they heal their bowel. The more money one has spent, and the more programs one has tried to get better or lose weight, the less time and money one may devote to this in the future, this program included.

But for this to work you have to devote time and money to it. You will fail if you only "try this" for a few months. You cannot reverse a lifetime of weakness in three months. I understand the reluctance to do this as you may rightly feel like this might just be another failure in your long list of them, and you don't want to waste your precious time and money on another failure.

Commit to a minimum of one year of this work. At this point, the majority of my clients have eliminated their fear of failing with this program; they really understand how this works and why it won't fail them; they have seen positive improvements and are committed to devoting more time to this process and finishing the healing work to the end.

I am 100% confident that this program will not fail you.

Be grateful there is an answer

Rather than focusing on how long this will take, be grateful that there is a way to heal your body and that you have found the right road to accomplish this. Many people spend years in psychotherapy before becoming healthier emotionally, so too should you approach this program.

You cannot focus solely on the end of this road. If you start off in China and desire to be in Nantucket, you need to enjoy the ride and see the arrival in Ohio as great progress rather than disappointment that you are not in Nantucket yet. Appreciate what is happening and what is possible.

When you heal your bowel and body, the "top of your pipe" heals first; the "dangerous" stuff gets fixed first. Often people don't even know there is a danger. The majority of cancer has been growing 10-20 years before it is detectable; 70% of your arteries could be clogged and you could be asymptomatic. Heart disease is called "the silent killer" for a reason. On the other hand, when your arteries are clearing up, this will occur "silently" as well. You will not feel this and can wrongly conclude that your body is not healing with this program. Trust that your body knows best and it is healing the scary, life-threatening stuff first. You will be focusing on the bottom of your pipe, but the top heals first, followed by the middle. So even if this takes time, you will at least *have* the time—i.e. will still likely be alive—to see this through to the end. I would rather spend two years healing my bowel and body than two years fighting cancer, and eventually dying from it much too young.

How long will my bowel stay healed? Will I have to re-do this program again?

I cannot guarantee that this will never have to be repeated, but I think the chances of this are extremely unlikely. There are 100 trillion bacteria in your bowel. Creating a healthy intestinal environment is an enormous feat. It is like building a twenty-four-room mansion. It takes a lot to ruin this house/upset this bacterial environment. I believe that many people leave this program with a bowel that is healthier than the one they came out into the world with. My bowel works better than I can ever remember.

When you are done you will have a brand new house, and a really strong one, too. This house is ruined by acids—from diet, stress, drugs, and the environment. With a strong bowel, many of these acids are avoided. When you heal your body, acidic foods are no longer desirable. It is therefore easy to avoid this cause of bowel breakdown. A healthy body will not crave sugar, alcohol, coffee, or chicken, for example—all foods that, over many years, cause your bowel to become less healthy.

Stress, another variable that can weaken your bowel, is still going to be present when you heal it, but even this is minimized when you heal your body. A healthy body is very empowering and creates a lot of security. The stress of getting a disease or of being unable to work due to fatigue or an illness, for example, is greatly minimized when you are healthy. Not having to worry about gaining weight is also a significant stress reducer!

As for drugs that can damage your bowel, these too will be dramatically reduced when you have healed your bowel and body. A healthy body will not need pain killers, antibiotics, or blood pressure regulators, etc.

A healthy body also has a balanced brain and blood chemistry. This eliminates the craving for acidic recreational drugs. I know.

Finally, environmental acids like pesticides, ammonia, and air pollution, can weaken your bowel too, but these too will be minimized after you heal your body. A healthy body will react to toxic odors, inspiring you to remove yourself from them. For example, when a new window was put into my basement a very toxic sealant was used. I immediately smelled this and didn't like it. The man installing the window was completely unaffected by it. I, on the other hand, found it disgusting, so I opened the window to air it out, closed the door to the basement and stayed out of it until the smell was gone. Not all of the environmental toxins are detectable, but a healthy body will detect a lot more than an unhealthy one, and this will help reduce your exposure to them.

In summary, when you are done healing your body and bowel, you will be "starting out" with a much stronger "house" than you had before this program. Also, variables that weaken your bowel will be minimized. You will have a much stronger house and a lot less rain hitting it than you did when you embarked on this program. If it took forty years to get where you were when you started this, and that was with an unhealthy bowel and 40 years of a high level of exposure to acids, then it may take 80 years to get back to that place, because you are starting off with a strong bowel and a significant reduction in acids entering your system. You may die before that happens.

In my experience, it is much easier to maintain bowel health than it is to achieve it.

Questions and Misunderstandings About Products That Heal Your Bowel

Numerous misunderstandings exist about the use of *Bowel Strength* and probiotics like acidophilus. I combat them daily. When these are clarified, ones chance of succeeding with this program is much higher. I continue to hear new ones and am sure that there are many more than I will address here, but hopefully I can provide you with enough clarification to keep you on the right road.

A quick reduction in symptoms does not mean you quickly healed your bowel

Often a client starts the *Bowel Strength* and quickly experiences less gas, or illness. It is sometimes interpreted as the result of quickly healing their bowel. This is understandable. Who wouldn't want to believe they are healthier than they really are, and that the answer to this will be quick and easy? This program is designed to be aggressive, but even in the best cases, healing takes time. If you feel better right away, it is because you are responding to one of the crutches in this product or to one of the crutches recommended in Chapters 8, 9, and 10.

Likewise, when people take acidophilus and feel a lot better right away, they often give the acidophilus all the credit, believing that it's possible to quickly heal their bowel. This is not true, and it is a belief that will reduce your success in healing your bowel and body.

When people take acidophilus and feel better right away, it's because they also made big changes to their diet or began using crutches at the same time. **It is not possible for acidophilus to immediately fix all of the holes in the roof that are the cause of your problem in the first place.**

I read an article in which a woman with Crohn's disease began taking acidophilus and in it she stated, "she believes the probiotics have helped, *along with the medication and restrictive diet.*" This shows my point exactly. In this case, the diet and medication are helping her symptoms the most. The acidophilus has not immediately helped. If you took her off the medication and restrictive diet crutches, I'm positive her symptoms would flare up again.

Bowel Strength and acidophilus heal your bowel. Envision thousands of holes in your roof and that every day that you take these products a few of these holes are being repaired. This will take time. If you start off with 10,000 holes and repair 1,000 of them, you are healthier and your roof is stronger, but you are still vulnerable to the rain that hits it; 9,000 holes are still left. To immediately protect your house from this rain you would need to avoid it or soak it up with a mop. **To immediately feel better or have better bowel movements, you will need to use a crutch, as described in Chapters 8, 9, and 10.**

Do not use *Bowel Strength* and acidophilus as crutches to treat symptoms

Many people have wrongly been advised to use acidophilus to treat symptoms as discussed above, including ear infections, yeast infections, gas, etc. Contrary to this popular advice, using acidophilus to treat a symptom can makes things worse, although in most cases, it simply doesn't work.

These products are healing, and as such, cannot immediately eliminate a symptom. You cannot immediately fix all of the holes in your roof that cause symptoms. In fact, *when you take acidophilus or Bowel Strength, there should be no immediate change in your symptoms or bowel movements. A lack of a reaction means you need it.* You are used to taking pills and immediately responding—because they are crutches—and this concept can be very different and confusing. However, it is an extremely important one to follow in order for this process to work.

Bowel Strength and acidophilus cannot immediately improve your stools

These products also cannot immediately improve the form of your stools. Likewise, do not use them as a laxative either. Over time your stools will become better formed and the frequency will improve, if that is an issue, but neither of these should happen immediately.

If the addition of any one of these products immediately produces more frequent stools, it means that you may be going too fast, and this is undesirable. Do not take more than you need.

People are commonly prescribed acidophilus when their stools are very loose. People who do not take acidophilus often experience a firmer stool following loose ones, because the looseness often motivates one to change their actions; actions that triggered the looseness in the first place. For example, if someone's bowel is weak, and a lot of acidic trash goes into it, their stools can get loose. This produces a lot of discomfort, and this discomfort usually makes one alter the acidic trash coming in. In other words, if you don't feel great you are less likely to eat, and less likely to drink or run around; actions that reduce the amount of acidity in your bowel.

If you have a firmer stool the day after taking acidophilus and you attribute it to the ingestion of this product, this is simply a product of misunderstanding, wishful thinking, or both. More importantly, if you make this wrong conclusion, your chance of failing to heal your bowel and body will increase.

Antibiotics do not kill all of your good bowel bacteria

Antibiotics are destructive to the good bacteria in your bowel; the ones that this program re-establishes. The problem is that many doctors and alternative health practitioners have been told to make a general recommendation of consuming two weeks worth of acidophilus, with no mention or attention given to the strength of the acidophilus used, to correct the damage done by antibiotic use.

In the twenty years that I have studied bowel health, ad nauseam, I have never once seen a study showing that the good bacteria that are killed off by antibiotics are automatically replaced by a two-week ingestion of a random amount of acidophilus.

This recommendation and misunderstanding is harmful for two reasons. One, it gives the impression that one can quickly, in two weeks time, reestablish good bacteria in their bowel. Two, many people have been led to believe that antibiotics kill off all of the good bacteria in your bowel. This is not true. If it were, millions of you would be dead!

Antibiotics do kill off some of the good bacteria, but for the vast majority of you who have taken them, an individualized, aggressive, long-term approach to the use of acidophilus is needed to heal your bowel. Also, it is harmful to believe that all of the good bacteria in your bowel are killed when you take antibiotics. This misunderstanding has led some people to be very fearful of using them. Antibiotics are not great for you, but sometimes the benefit far outweighs the damage caused by them. There are times when they should be taken. They can be life saving and/or stop dangerous cases of diarrhea caused by bacterial infections. For others, they are the only things that can "get them back to work or back on their feet." My clients are advised to try goldenseal and/or colloidal silver to fight bacterial infections if they have one, but to never put themselves in harms way if they are really ill, and to take antibiotics if necessary.

The bowel-healing program presented here will far compensate for any damage done by using antibiotics.

Likewise, never use *Bowel Strength* or acidophilus in place of an antibiotic. When you use these to strengthen your bowel, you will not get bacterial infections, but these products cannot *immediately* destroy germs. Only antibiotics or natural crutches, like colloidal silver and goldenseal, have the ability to immediately kill germs.

Bowel Strength and garlic breath and/or indigestion

Roughly 5% of my clients complain of garlic breath or discomfort after swallowing these pills. This process does not need to be uncomfortable, so if this happens to you, switch to powdered acidophilus instead. On the other hand, if the garlic does not bother you, or your loved ones, continue with it. This reaction will eventually go away. I surmise that individuals with an inflamed esophagus are the ones that react most negatively to this product. Healing your bowel will eventually eliminate the inflammation causing this problem, and eventually this reaction will stop. Indigestion after swallowing the pills or garlic breath does not mean that this product is too strong.

Programs That Do Not Heal Your Bowel, Although You May Be Wrongly Led to Believe Otherwise

Laxatives, even natural ones, do not heal

A product that is taken to stimulate a bowel movement is called a laxative. Generally, these work by stimulating your bowel to contract more intensely, forcing the contents inside to move out. Some of the most commonly used, natural laxatives are cascara sagrada, senna, aloe vera, buckthorn bark, and rhubarb. Over the counter laxatives often contain these ingredients as well, but may also contain synthetic stimulants as well. These products do not heal your bowel bacteria, which need to be healthy to have frequent bowel movements naturally!

Because everyone likes to believe they can fix their body overnight and because most people think that a product that immediately improves the frequency of their bowel movements has done that, the majority of bowel supplements and colon cleansers contain laxatives. It keeps people coming back to buy many more of these products.

Psyllium and other fibers, including dietary fiber, do not heal your bowel

Fiber does not heal your bowel bacteria either. If your bacterial levels are unhealthy, the addition of extra fiber to your diet can cause gas, diarrhea, discomforts, and other problems that can easily lead one to avoid it. If this happens when you increase your fiber intake, reduce or stop it until your bowel bacteria are healthier. *You will regain your health and lose weight much more quickly if you heal your bowel bacteria prior to increasing your fiber intake. (High fiber foods include bran, whole grains, beans, raw vegetables including salads, and nuts.)*

Fiber has been emphasized as a laxative product with benefit primarily for those with constipation. This is untrue. Fiber helps you eliminate the acidity from your blood. Fiber helps move this acidity into your bowel. Excess acids in your blood cause cholesterol levels to rise, blood sugar levels to rise, and your weight to go up. As such, I am a big fan of fiber, but do not confuse it with *Bowel Strength* or acidophilus. Some studies claim that higher fiber consumption eliminates certain toxins, but this is not true. **Fiber moves toxins from your blood into your bowel, but it is a healthy bowel—as you are creating in this program-- that eliminates the toxins, not the fiber itself.**

197

Fiber should not be treated like a laxative. If you get a laxative effect from it—it makes your bowels more frequent right away, this is usually a sign that your bowel bacterial environment is unhealthy, and you should pay attention to healing that instead. If you do not respect this, the healing of your body will take a long time, if at all. You will be very uncomfortable and likely to quit the process altogether.

Nystatin, caprylic acid, anti-fungals, zappers, and other products that do not heal

A common but wrong approach that is used for bowel health is the administration of herbs or medications that kill off bad bacteria, fungus, and yeast in your bowel. Any medication, such as Nystatin, that kills off yeast is toxic and weakens your bowel further. In the meantime, there is a short-term period where one feels better because the bad guys have been killed. But the bad bacteria eventually return, and at a higher level than before, because of the weaker bowel caused by the drug.

While natural supplements and products that kill off Candida, fungus, yeast, and parasites—like anti-fungals and zappers, are not toxic and do not cause things to get worse in the long run, they also do nothing to fix the cause of the problem in the first place, either. If you have holes in your trashcan, trash will leak out onto the ground, which will attract bugs. *Killing the bugs gets rid of them for a while, but they will eventually come back because killing them did nothing to fix the holes in the trashcan.* The leaky trashcan will continue to leak and the bugs will eventually find their way back. The holes in the trashcan must be fixed, as this program does.

Programs that recommend products that kill Candida and yeast describe a side effect that they term "die-off." This happens when you kill the Candida and yeast faster than you can eliminate the toxic by-products of them and it is uncomfortable, not very effective in the long run, and unnecessary.

If you feel bad, something is wrong. This will not happen if you follow this program of healing your bowel.

Homeostatic soil organisms (HSOs)

A recent bestselling health book recommends the use of homeostatic soil organisms for improving bowel health. I have never used these in my practice, but I highly question their ability to heal your bowel. This skepticism comes from a comment from the author that states that this product helps to create a reservoir of extra antibodies that support immune function, but that this reservoir "diminishes when HSO ingestion ends." *If something improves only when you are taking it, then you have treated the symptoms of the problem and not the cause.* This is one definition of a crutch, and crutches do not heal. Given this information, I would not compare HSOs to *Bowel Strength* or acidophilus, products that I have used for over 16 years to help clients heal their bowel and body; products that do not, and in fact cannot, be taken long-term.

L-glutamine, etc.

L-glutamine is a popular supplement for aiding in the repair of a damaged bowel, damage that is caused by excess acidity and a weakened bacterial environment. I have seen people misled into thinking they can magically heal their bowel "overnight" by using it, but I have never seen this happen. There is no magic, quick fix for healing your bowel.

Likewise, you will be able to find a number of other products that have similar, yet not the same, ingredients as *Bowel Strength*. Watch out for these. I have checked out many over the years and so far, all of these other products are geared more to treating the symptoms of an unhealthy bowel than healing it. Some of these are a little less expensive, but in the long run, you will actually pay much more. These products take much longer to heal the bowel, so you will need them for much longer than *Bowel Strength*. This means that you will spend the same or more money in the long run. You will also need to take other crutches longer if it takes a long time to heal your bowel, making it more likely that you will spend more.

Just because a program includes probiotics or similar herbs as *Bowel Strength,* does not mean it is healing your bowel

The majority of the bowel products are crutches that do not heal your bowel. For example, a product may contain a very small amount of acidophilus with a large amount of a laxative and anti-gas herb. This produces immediate gas reduction and an immediate increase in the frequency of one's elimination, but the acidophilus—the part that heals your bowel so that the cause of gas and poor elimination is addressed—is insufficient to heal.

I have seen many clients who were falsely led into believing that they had healed their bowel because they took bowel supplements and/or colon cleansers.

A recent advertisement, from a supplement company marketing a product for the bowel, touted a product that consisted of a 10-day kit that, it was claimed, "restores natural gut flora." But this product also includes many "crutches." Here is a fact. You cannot restore your gut bacteria in only ten days. Many of you will assume that you did, as the crutches in the product can immediately affect your bowels; it contains a laxative that makes you go more often, and everyone wants to believe that this means they healed their bowel.

Finally, if probiotics are taken with a restrictive, low carbohydrate diet, it is the "crutch-like" effect of this diet that is helping you feel and look better in the short-term, not the probiotics. Worst of all, not only are you driving down the road at 1 mph, but the high protein diet, which damages your bowel further, throws you into reverse so that you are *not even driving forward and* healing your bowel, but making it less healthy.

Any product that claims a quick or inexpensive fix

It is factually impossible to heal your bowel "overnight," and anyone or any product, like the one mentioned above, that claims to do this will definitely end up failing to deliver on this promise. In the meantime, you have wasted your precious time and money heading down the wrong road.

Recently I saw an article stating that the makers of Dannon yogurt have had a class action suit filed against their claim that one of their yogurt products will fix digestive problems in three weeks. I am thrilled that this action has been taken; it should be. Anyone filing these claims is correct. Not only can you not heal your bowel in three weeks, you most certainly cannot do it with a product like yogurt that contains relatively minute amounts of probiotics.

The damage that this false marketing and advertising campaigns create is not erased by this lawsuit. Most of you would not have known about it had you not read about it here. The vast majority of you will have this commercial in your head, the one promising a very quick healing of your bowel. This expectation, along with all of the other false advertising you have ever heard, leads you down the wrong road over and over again.

Likewise, I anticipate a slew of products marketed in response to this book that claim to cost much less than the products I am promoting. **You get what you pay for.** *Bowel Strength* and the probiotics I recommend work because of the ingredients in them, and they are not cheap. I have seen clients fall for products that they perceived—due to clever marketing on a company's part—to be equal to these, and this has always been a disaster. If you fall for a less expensive product, it will take much longer to heal your bowel and you will end up paying much more money in the long run. If you can find inexpensive crutches, similar to those listed in Chapter 10, that is great, but do not attempt this program with any product except for *Bowel Strength* or a very high quality, powerful probiotic, preferably the one I suggested from ProThera.

Enemas and colonics

On her show in the winter 2006, Oprah stated that people ask about colonics all the time. A woman in the audience described her experience with colonics, in which she spent a couple hundred dollars for the procedures and saw no weight loss as a result, which was her original intent in pursuing colonics.

The greatest value of enemas and colonics is the elimination of uncomfortable gas and bloating. The promise of healing your bowel and body, and of eliminating vast quantities of waste and fat, is one that is overstated and highly misrepresented.

Twenty years ago when I was disabled with my autoimmune disease, I read a book on the colon and it made sense to me that the elimination of waste would help heal my body. For as long as I could remember, I had very infrequent bowel movements, approximately once every three or four days, and when I did go, my stools were small and hard. I had no awareness at the time that this was harmful and no knowledge of what was normal. Mostly, I was glad that I didn't go often as I found it embarrassing to use the bathroom in places other than my home, and I was hardly ever home.

The first time I have any recollection of my bowel movements was at age eleven. I was hospitalized with appendicitis and a couple days after the operation, the surgeon asked me if I had had a bowel movement. I didn't even know what he meant by that! So I lied and said yes. Truth is, I hadn't. I never forgot that question, though. It was the first time the concept of pooping was brought up to me and I got that it had some importance. Later on, I was a little more aware of my elimination, although I never knew if it was healthy, and I never did anything about it.

So when I was very ill and still constipated I decided this must be changed. I had read enough to understand that it was not healthy not to go every day.

Eighty colonics and over four hundred enemas later

I went to a colon therapist and had many colonics, thinking that I would be eliminating large amounts of toxins from my body. The sessions were expensive and uncomfortable, but I thought they were helping me heal my body and I was willing to do whatever it took to accomplish that. I did at least

201

eighty colonics. After each one my stomach was flatter, as I had eliminated a large quantity of gas, but I didn't feel a lot better. Therapists claim that some people feel lighter, have more energy, and are calmer, but I never did. And I had to constantly fight with the therapist against purchasing a multitude of supplements from him, usually ones that were part of his latest get-rich, multi-level-marketing scheme.

In addition to the colonics, I did at least 400 enemas at home. I thought this gave me an inexpensive way to quickly and consistently continue the elimination of toxins from my body. Again, I felt no noticeable improvement in my health afterwards, but I was sold on their ability to help heal my body.

After some 80 colonics and some 400 enemas, my bowel function was exactly the same as it was before I started! I still had infrequent, hard stools. The only thing that changed my elimination and made it healthy was the program that I am teaching you here. This program also healed my body, something the enemas and colonics never did.

Many years ago some progressive thinkers caught on to the notion that a healthy colon and a healthy body went hand in hand. How enemas and colonics evolved from there I do not know, but like many things in life, the use of these two modalities was a start in the right direction, rather than the right direction itself.

The trash is reabsorbed

When your bowel bacteria are unhealthy and/or there is an excess of acidity in your bowel, acids are inefficiently converted into a stool. What is not formed into a stool is rapidly reabsorbed back into the rest of your body. Here is the major problem of colonics and enemas. The waste that you are supposed to be eliminating is rarely present in your bowel to be eliminated when the colonic is done. It has already been reabsorbed, and the colonic can't get to it when this has happened. In other words, your body throws some trash into the trashcan, but when it gets to the trashcan, if it can't fit because the trashcan is too small, the trash goes back into your house where it came from. Then along comes a hose to clean out the trashcan, but there is no trash in there to rinse out. It all went back into the house! When I had all of my colonics done I saw some formed stool come out, but I saw a lot more gas eliminated and a lot of brown liquid as well, a sign that the acids in my bowel were not getting formed up and were being reabsorbed back into my body.

Proper formation of a stool and the efficient elimination of it require healthy bowel bacteria. Enemas and colonics do nothing to strengthen your bowel bacteria. Finally, the gas that an enema eliminates can make one feel better and less bloated temporarily, but it does nothing to prevent the formation of gas in the first place.

Many colon therapists also recommend strict wheat and dairy free diets as well as numerous supplements, so is it the colonic or the diet and supplements that are really helping? I believe that any symptomatic relief one achieves after the colonic is primarily due to these.

A popular doctor on television said that colonics are not needed because the body cleanses itself in one to two days. With perfect bowel health this is true, but who watching this show has perfect bowel health? Not many people, if anyone at all! Your body cannot cleanse itself unless your bowel bacteria are strong and acids are finding their way into it. For the majority of you, one or both of these conditions do not exist, and vast quantities of acids accumulate in your body as a result.

Enemas and colonics can release the old, encrusted waste on the wall of the colon, but it will build right back up if your bowel is not healed. They can also help discharge yeast and parasites. But again, these will come back if your bowel is not healed. When you get rid of the waste in your intestinal tract, the mucus lining will no longer be needed to protect your bowel from toxins, and this lining will get shed *without colonics*. You absorb nutrients better when the mucus lining is gone. *Healing your bowel with this program will eliminate this build-up on your colon wall, eliminate yeast, toxins, and parasites, and do this in a way that is permanent and complete.* "Internal cleansing" with colonics and herbs would not be needed if your bowel were healthy and as a result, kept clean on a day-to-day basis, naturally.

The Definition of a Bowel That Has Been Healed

Other people and programs claim that symptoms have gone away after healing the bowel, but to date, I have not found any proof that any of these programs have actually done that. A mother with an autistic child, who is involved in an autism support group that has raised millions of dollars, claimed that her son's autism improved after the *elimination of environmental toxins* and the healing of his bowel If his bowel were healed, he could be exposed to environmental toxins without his symptoms flaring up. When I was ill I had to move out of a new house because I had a severe reaction to the chemicals in the new paint and carpeting. These chemicals no longer affect me.

An article in our local paper reported on a woman with lupus who had reduced her symptoms by healing her bowel, but she also followed a *strict diet* and was taking *medications* as well.

Can you claim that you healed your bowel when other variables are in the picture? Would these people have improved had they followed a strict diet, used medications, and/or avoided environmental toxins, for example, but not taken any products to help the bowel? Just because you take a product and feel better, does it mean that the product helped, when other products were introduced at the same time? If you need $3 to buy something and you give someone $4, the extra $1 did not contribute to your ability to buy that item.

A recent best-selling book that claims to heal the bowel promotes a high protein, low carbohydrate diet with the consumption of good quality sugars, salt, vinegar, etc. It is based on the Bible, but the Bible can be interpreted numerous ways. The author says that fiber from carbohydrates causes intestinal disease and he personally won't eat bran because he can't eat it with his Chron's disease! He says he healed his bowel, but this can't be true. If he had, he could eat fiber and carbohydrates without experiencing discomfort. Also, not once in the book is there a description of ideal bowel movements.

There is a story of a woman who followed this diet who took the supplements and described her three days off the diet this way: "I was able to see and feel the negative results of those choices within hours (stomach cramps, bloating, headaches, brain fog and fatigue). It is almost like these foods are toxic to my body…I am literally allergic to particular foods…my body just can't process them." She then goes on to say, "I'm sure my bowels are being cleansed as well, because I believe it." *Believing something does not mean it is happening.*

A new client came in today with a history of decades worth of bowel problems and she said she healed it because her chiropractor gave her a supplement called "Gut Support" and her symptoms are better. She is ingesting digestive enzymes daily and avoiding dairy, wheat, and sugar and eating a high-protein diet. This is not the definition of a healed bowel!

Of the examples I have given above, none of the people claiming to heal their bowels could answer, "yes" to situations described below.

If you really healed your bowel the following would be true

-- You could eat whatever you wanted without bowel or other symptoms flaring up.

-- You could expose yourself to mental or environmental stressors without symptoms flaring up.

-- You would have ideal elimination no matter what you ate or did.

-- You could completely stop all supplements without symptoms flaring up.

Not qualified to give advice on healing your bowel

Most of the clients I see who have experience with alternative health have never worked with a practitioner who has focused on their bowel. When they have, it has always been very poorly and ineffectively done. I find it especially humorous, and pathetic, when a practitioner pretends to be helping your bowel, but never has discussions with you about the form of your stools. You cannot possibly help someone heal his or her bowel without this knowledge. I call these practitioners the great pretenders. **If you see a practitioner who says he is helping you with your bowel but then never asks about the form of your stools, find someone else.** Also, if **a practitioner claims to have a way to quickly heal your bowel, they are wrong. There are ways to quickly treat the symptoms of your bowel, like laxatives that make you go more often, but there is no quick way to heal your bowel.**

Several years ago I saw a client who three years prior had worked with a local doctor who bills himself as an alternative doctor. He offered her a quick fix. He gave her the same product I do to heal her bowel, but he also gave her numerous other supplement crutches, because that is what all doctors do, even all of the alternative doctors I have ever met or read about. She believed that she had healed her bowel with him, and he agreed, because she felt better.

Feeling better does not mean that your bowel has healed. Taking a lot of crutches can help you feel better. When you take numerous products you cannot claim that one helped. In this case, the doctor gave her a great product to help heal her bowel, but he did not know how to use it. He thought it worked immediately, like other crutches. And he gave her a very small, insufficient amount for a very short, insufficient length of time. The choice of product was good, but it was never used correctly and it was not the reason she felt better. When she came into my office her bowel was extremely unhealthy. It had not been healed. By the way, if it *had* been, three years later she could not have entered my office with an extremely unhealthy one. It takes much longer than three years to weaken your bowel. **Just because a practitioner or author talks about the importance of the bowel does not mean he or she knows how to heal it.**

Years ago I had a client who took the *Bowel Strength* to her acupuncturist and she told her it was a bad product. The acupuncturist also told her that she has had colitis, an inflammatory bowel problem, for twenty years. You are crazy if you take advice about how to heal your bowel from someone who has had colitis for twenty years. Colitis can only occur when your bowel is unhealthy. **If you take advice about healing your bowel, make sure it is from someone with a healthy bowel, not someone with a bowel problem like colitis!**

Don't ask your alternative health practitioner for his or her opinion

Would you come to me for advice on how to fix your car? I sure hope not, because this is something I do not know how to do and am not qualified to comment on. If you see a mechanic and he suggests a program for fixing your car, do not "run it by me" to see if it makes sense. And if I did pretend to know how to do this and commented on this mechanic's program, I hope you would lose respect for me for doing so.

With the same mentality in mind, do not ask your acupuncturist, doctor, naturopath, chiropractor—*or any other practitioner who depends on crutches and does not know how to heal your bowel or body*—if they think this program is good. They are not qualified to comment on it, good or bad. And they are disrespecting you and me when they do so. But only you are at risk of being harmed by this. (The people working at the health food store are not qualified to comment on it either.)

If you want to heal your body and need some support for what we are doing here, you will have a hard time finding a book or practitioner who can help you. This is the sad truth. I have done my best to support you as much as I can with this book and follow-ups to it. If you think you have found a practitioner who can help you, ask questions, the right questions. For example, **if you are still tempted to ask your naturopath about the *Bowel Strength*, for example, then also ask your naturopath to describe his stools in detail to you.** If they do not match the ideal bowel description given in Chapter 6, then this is not the person to be taking advice from in healing your bowel. If their bowel movements sound good, then ask about their diet. If chicken, turkey, eggs, and/or fish are consumed more than one time a day and they limit carbohydrates, then they are eating a high protein diet, and that means their bowel is unhealthy, even if their stools are good. Also, if they have to avoid wheat or dairy, they have an unhealthy bowel. No further questions are needed to confirm that this is not the person you want to get advice from on healing your bowel. There are other good questions to ask too, however, my bet is that these alone will steer you in the right direction, because I bet that none of the people you ask will be able to give you the right answer.

Signs that a diet or supplement program won't heal your bowel properly

1. Individualized recommendations are not made for the use of the supplements.

2. There is no discussion about your stools, especially as pertains to their form.

3. There is an implied "quick fix" of your bowel using the supplements or following the diet.

4. A high protein diet is recommended, i.e., chicken, beef, eggs, turkey and/ or fish are consumed 2-3x/day and high carbohydrate foods—like breads and pastas—are limited.

5. The program requires long-term dependence on a strict diet or supplements to maintain symptomatic results or weight loss.

A tough mind-set to change

It is very difficult to change the way you have thought about and approached health. I suspect that doctors, naturopaths, chiropractors, acupuncturists, and other practitioners who have been trained to treat symptoms with crutches will have a very difficult time changing this mentality and using these bowel-healing products correctly, too.

In consideration of this, if you need extra support during this process, I recommend two avenues: One, re-read this book many times. It contains a lot of new, complex information that will take a while to sink in. Look for follow-ups to this book too. They will contain a wealth of additional information to support you. Two, contact me at donna@ThisWorksCrutchesDont.com and we can work together individually, or if you prefer and/or if I'm not available, log onto my blog at www.ThisWorksCrutchesDont.blogspot.com.

When to seek professional help

The maximum quantities of acidophilus and *Bowel Strength* that I have listed are much less than the maximums I use in my office with clients. For many of you, these maximums will be sufficient enough to produce results in a reasonable period of time and without much complication. But for many others, the complexity of your health and/or weakness in your bowel will necessitate a more individualized and more aggressive program.

If you have reached the maximum level recommended and /or are encountering a number of confusing or complex issues along this path, please contact me at donna@ThisWorksCrutchesDont.com to schedule an appointment.

Some clients who have benefited from a much more aggressive and individualized program are those with ADD, arthritis, autism, alcohol and drug addictions, autoimmune disorders, cancer, celiac, Chron's disease, colitis, diabetes, elevated cholesterol levels, heart disease, hemorrhoids, hepatitis, and severe food and/or environmental allergies. These conditions reflect an extremely weak bowel and a very complex health condition that are best approached individually. Nevertheless, if you can get started with understanding the concepts I have explained and start incorporating the ideas herein, you will be miles ahead of those who are not doing this program and heading in the wrong direction.

The main reason I almost didn't write this book

The greatest challenge I have had in writing this book is the fact that it can't be approached as a simple "one program for everyone" recommendation. When I work with clients our consultations can be very complex and often require a lot of time, experimentation and feedback. I thought, "How do I accomplish this in a book?"

I have come to accept two things. One, you need and deserve to read and learn the information that I have. Ultimately, I couldn't let this stop me from writing this book. And two, driving slowly down the right road is still far preferable than driving slowly, or fast, down the wrong road. I absolutely cannot provide you with all of the information that I know and make the same aggressive recommendations to you through this book as I can with you individually, but hopefully I can get you thinking, give you hope, and lead you in the right direction. That is my ultimate goal in writing this book.

Chapter Eight

Healing Your Body

When you heal your bowel with the instructions given in Chapter 7, the rest of your body will heal too. When you make space in your trashcan, the trash in the rest of your house will take advantage of this and move into this space to be eliminated. When you heal your bowel, the accumulated acidity in your other organs that causes symptoms, illness and disease, addictions, and weight gain, will enter your bowel to be eliminated.

If "it" doesn't result in a positive exit of acidity from your body, then "it" is not really healing you.

Healing should be comfortable; if it is not, you are doing something wrong.

Most diets, supplements and alternative programs rely on crutches and crutches do not heal; therefore, the following concepts and experiences will be new to the majority of you.

This chapter explains what to expect as you heal your body. This information constitutes a vital "map" that will help you succeed as you travel down this healing road. This information is some of the most important that a client needs in order to succeed. I encourage them to re-read this section at least monthly, and I encourage you to do the same. Read it more frequently if you are ever confused or concerned about your symptoms or how your body is reacting to the supplements you are taking. **A misunderstanding of the healing process is one of the main reasons why an individual will fail to achieve their health and weight potential.**

An Interpretation of Your Symptoms as You Heal

During this healing program, you will not look or feel worse due to the program itself if you follow the directions carefully in the last chapter on healing your bowel, and in this chapter on healing your body.

It is incredibly important that you "blame the right thing" if you are not feeling well or gaining weight while you are healing your body. Even when I work directly with clients, they frequently blame the wrong thing, and we spend some unnecessary time getting them back on track. In some cases, a client blames the wrong thing and gets completely off track, failing to heal their body as a result.

There are only three possible reasons why you may experience an increase or occurrence of a symptom or your weight during this program. While these are not due to this healing program, they can occur during it, and your understanding of them will help make this process a fast, easy, comfortable, and successful one.

#1--You reduce your protein intake too soon

A nutritional program that is cleansing is one that is very low in protein, high in fiber, and high in carbohydrates/glucose. This stimulates your cells to release acids into your blood, acids that otherwise set the stage for disease and illness. **When you switch from an unhealthy high protein diet to a healthy low protein diet, uncomfortable reactions and weight gain can occur due to the release of acids into your bloodstream at a rate faster than your bowel can eliminate them.** Many books that were written decades ago described some of these reactions as "healing reactions." They were described as desirable and people were told to grin and bear it. I strongly disagree.

It is admirable if you want to quickly improve the healthfulness of your diet by eating less protein, but it will get you in trouble because you cannot quickly improve the health of your bowel. **If you make this change too quickly, you will look and feel worse and there is an extremely slim chance that you will continue on this path and this program, and a very large chance you will fail to heal your body. Therefore, it is vitally important that you do not immediately reduce the amount of protein that you eat. (Do not eat less meat, chicken, turkey, eggs, fish, etc.)** Even the smallest reduction in your protein intake can trigger health and weight symptoms if it occurs prior to a significant healing of your bowel. For example, if you usually eat two eggs for breakfast and reduce this to one, you are setting yourself up to feel and look worse. Review your diet and if you have reduced your protein intake, raise it back to previous levels and see if that improves your symptoms/weight.

It can take three months or one year or longer before your bowel is strong enough to better eliminate the acids that a lower protein diet "stirs up."

Most programs and diets do not heal your body. Most programs incorporate a high protein diet and you *can* make drastic changes towards this without any discomfort. This program heals, which is why weight loss becomes permanent and eventually effortless, and it is why you will eliminate all chances of future illness. But it is also why dietary changes on this program need to be slow and gradual. *Making sudden changes will result in more discomfort and a higher chance of failure.*

The most important ingredient for successfully healing your body is not a radical shift in your diet. It is patience. Your bowel will heal if your diet is not perfect; the best way to get to a healthy diet, in fact, is to heal your bowel first. The best way to minimize these reactions is to be patient with your body and this program. Do not force too many new changes too fast. Trust your body. When your bowel is strong enough to eliminate acids more efficiently, you will automatically and naturally desire less protein. Waiting for this to happen is very different from forcing it to happen. As your bowel become stronger, the elimination of acids from your blood will occur rapidly and comfortably.

#2--More rain hits your roof and/or you yank the tarp off of it too soon

You have *current* symptoms and excess weight due to an inability to eliminate acids efficiently. These symptoms can become exacerbated if you are exposed to more acids than usual.

The most significant sources of dietary acids that can cause a symptom(s) or weight gain are: sugar, salt, coffee, alcohol, soda, refined carbohydrates like bagels and pizza, and any food that you may be allergic to. If consumption of *any* of these foods have increased recently, then your increased symptoms are likely due to this and not to the supplements or healing. If you have been eating out at restaurants more often, you may feel worse due to the excessive acidic salt in much of this food, for example. **If it rains harder, blame the rain for making your house wet, not the men fixing the holes on your roof. Do not blame the *Bowel Strength* or probiotics.**

In addition to "dietary rain," excess stress, travel, significant changes in climate, humidity, altitude, a disturbance in your sleep resulting in less than normal, over-exertion with exercise, a massage, dental fillings or any medical procedure, exposure to toxic chemicals in the environment or elsewhere (like new paint and carpet, for example), can also create more rain that triggers symptoms prior to all of the holes being fixed in your roof. Mental stressors are often obvious while environmental ones can be less so.

Once I received a phone call from a client whose son has Tourett's. He has been doing really well on this program, and his symptoms have reduced noticeably. We are still healing his bowel, however. This child's mother does a great job of protecting him from acids, so there is usually little rain hitting his roof. But five days prior, the thunderstorms came. While she was out of town, his dad took him out to eat every night at a restaurant chain that uses enormous amounts of salt, he had dental work done, and he was exposed to a flu virus at school that he caught. His symptoms came back. His bowel is not strong enough yet to handle this much rain. While this type of occurrence is always very hard for a person, it needs to be assessed realistically in order to succeed with this program. This child had a flare-up of his symptoms, which is simply a measure of the need to continue healing his bowel. This was actually an invaluable experience, because the mother wrongly and dangerously thought that because his symptoms had improved so much, his bowel was almost fixed. When the thunderstorm came, it showed her that this was not the case, yet. He is now doing well again and back on an aggressive amount of acidophilus to continue healing his bowel, and he will be much healthier as a result.

When you heal, the disappearance of a symptom does not mean that your bowel is completely healed and that your symptoms will be gone forever, yet. When the supplements you are taking for your bowel, the *Bowel Strength* and acidophilus, become too strong, *then* your bowel is healed and your symptoms will stay away. Until then, even if your symptoms are better, realize that you are still vulnerable to the rain that hits your roof. Do not misunderstand, misinterpret, or become discouraged by your symptoms if they do reappear prior to completing this process. **The presence of symptoms does not mean that you are not healing, doing something wrong, or taking the wrong dose of the supplements.**

If there are holes in your roof, every time it rains, your house gets wet. These holes cannot all be repaired overnight; your bowel and body cannot become healthier overnight either. As you become healthier, you will continue to experience symptoms until your body is completely healed, yet they will gradually diminish in occurrence and intensity. As your roof becomes stronger, your house gets less wet when it rains. As your body becomes healthier, it will be able to withstand acids without a reaction.

When a symptom occurs or increases due to more rain hitting your roof, it has nothing to do with this program. This program did not cause it. On the contrary, this program is needed to prevent this from happening in the future. This program is needed to fix your roof so you don't react poorly to the rain hitting it. All of the rain cannot be avoided, and it is far better to create a stronger roof than it is to try to always avoid the rain! Even if you could avoid this rain, a house with a strong roof with no holes in it that is rained on will last much longer than a house with a very weak roof, that hardly gets rained on.

Likewise, if you start this program with a strong tarp covering the holes on your roof and remove this before the holes are repaired, your house will get wet. If you start this program and rely on exercise to keep your weight down, and stop this before you have healed your bowel and body, you will gain weight. If chiropractic adjustments keep your back pain-free and you stop these at the beginning of this program, your back pain will return. These reactions have nothing to do with this program, either. They would have happened anyway. They are also another reason why healing your bowel and body are important, so that you can get rid of these crutches and not feel or look worse when you do. Remember, diets, drugs, exercise, vitamins, and physical modalities like acupuncture are crutches that make you look and feel better when your bowel and body are unhealthy. *If you change or eliminate one of these that you have been relying on at the beginning of this program, blame the elimination of the crutch, and not the Bowel Strength or probiotics, for causing your symptoms or weight increase.*

Yesterday a young woman with breast cancer tried to wrongly blame the *Bowel Strength* for causing her increase in acne. After making this accusation, she informed me that, as a result of her diagnosis, she had stopped using the chemicals on her face that she had been using to keep her skin clear. She removed a tarp and wanted to blame the supplements instead! She is very intelligent and I could not figure out how she could not "get the obvious." After sleeping on it, I realized that it has nothing to do with intelligence or common sense; she is simply driven by fear, as many cancer patients are.

I'll state it again. One of my main objectives with this book is to educate and empower you so that your unjustified fears are minimized and eliminated. Fear is the greatest deterrent to success in healing your bowel and body and attaining the success that is possible, and that you deserve.

#3--You drive too fast

You will be uncomfortable if you take the *Bowel Strength* or probiotics incorrectly, which almost always means that the amount you are taking is too strong and your stools have become loose because of it. Not all of these situations when your stools become loose are because of this, however. Make sure that you follow all of the instructions in the last chapter carefully. Not only will you be more uncomfortable if you take these incorrectly, but it will also take longer than necessary to lose weight and feel great.

In summary, these supplements are healing, and healing supplements need to be used respectively. If you are feeling worse, it is advisable that you stop these for a few days to see if they are causing a problem. If they are, you will know within a day or two. If you feel and/or look better after stopping them, re-introduce them in a few days to be sure they were really the cause of the problem. If adding them back re-aggravates your body, they are probably to blame, in which case you should reduce them to half the amount that you were taking before. If stopping them does not noticeably improve things in a few days, they are not causing your problem.

When you heal your bowel, the old, weak, toxic, acidic cells and unhealthy bacterium in it will be replaced with new, strong, healthy ones. When you try to heal too quickly, these old cells get replaced more rapidly than your body can handle them. They will get reabsorbed into your blood, lymphatic, and nervous systems and make you feel bad. If you start ripping all of the kitchen cabinets off of your kitchen walls and there is no space for them in the trashcans out front, your kitchen will look like a mess, and probably your family room and living room too, as you try to find a place for all that trash. **Being inpatient and trying to go too fast always backfires.** This can and should be avoided completely as long as you follow the directions on healing your bowel in Chapter 7.

Healing Reactions: Two Examples of Positive Healing Symptoms

During this process there are two categories of healing symptoms that you may experience. Both are positive signs that you are healing and neither is uncomfortable. More so, they can be completely misunderstood and misinterpreted, and this leaves one vulnerable to failing to heal their body. After you read these two scenarios, come back and re-read this section again every month or so. This way, when they occur, you will be ready for them and understand what they mean and what to do about them.

First example: symptoms become less frequent but they do not immediately disappear

Symptoms can immediately "disappear" only when you are treating them with crutches. They do not immediately disappear when you are healing your bowel and body and getting to the cause of them. In the long run, they will disappear and stay gone effortlessly. This is a far cry from the results you get when you simply treat them, which is inevitable failure, the development of new illnesses, and a shortened lifespan.

When you successfully heal your bowel and body, you will experience a gradual reduction in the frequency and severity of your symptoms. On the other hand, you are given instructions for using crutches in Chapter 10, and these will immediately reduce your symptoms and improve your bowel movements, but do not confuse this with healing, and do not interpret this to mean that you have quickly healed your bowel and body.

During the healing process, your body will release stored-up acidity from your cells and dump it into your organs of elimination. This is very positive and you will experience an improvement in your health and weight as a result. When you unplug the bottom of your pipe (organs of elimination), the acidity that was stuck in the middle and top will be released into the space that was just cleared away at the bottom. This is a wonderful thing that helps save your life, as trash at the top of your pipe is very harmful and undesirable. If your body can release it into your bowel because it is healthier, it will do so.

For example, after some time has been spent healing their bowel, a person who has had bloating and unformed stools for the last twenty years will find that a few days go by where the bloating is significantly better and the form of their stools has improved. Immediately following this, they may experience bloating and loose stools again. *When an original symptom improves but becomes unstable again, it can occur because your body is healing.*

The improvement in the form of your stools means that your body is eliminating a lot more acids than before, but it also sets your body up to release some accumulated acids into this area. *When an original symptom gets better, it may be followed by a period of the symptom returning again, until all of the old acids have been moved out.* In this example of a healing reaction, the original symptom is showing overall improvement; it is occurring with less frequency than it did before, and its return is no more uncomfortable than it was before.

Another way to explain this is that if your trashcan gets stronger and some space is cleared in it as a result, your kitchen may respond and throw some trash into it, which results in a cleaner kitchen but a trashcan that previously had space in it, becoming full again. As long as there is trash in the kitchen that needs to be thrown away, there will be days that the "trashcan is full."

This is not a negative experience. On the contrary, during these reactions, you are becoming healthier. The only time that this is interpreted as negative is when someone experiences the initial signs of improvement and is mentally disappointed when the improvement does not continue uninterrupted. *It is only after all of the old accumulated acidity has been eliminated that a symptom may be gone forever.*

If your symptoms fluctuate on this program it means that either there are fluctuations in the amount of rain hitting your roof (from diet, stress, etc), or that your body is healing and acids from other parts of your body are moving through your system to be eliminated.

You are used to crutches, and this can cause you to wrongly interpret these reactions and fail to heal your body. When you take a drug to lower your blood pressure, for example, and it does just that, you would rightly be concerned if at some point your blood pressure became elevated again while taking it. The medication is treating the symptom of high blood pressure and the return of that symptom means the drug may not be working anymore and may need to be increased. Your crutch is failing you.

During this process, the appearance of a symptom does not mean that the process is not working. As the frequency and intensity of an existing symptom improves, you will know that this process is proving beneficial to you, and that you are becoming healthier.

Second example: the scenery changes as you drive towards your optimum health and weight potential

As you heal, your symptoms will change as your body becomes healthier. **New symptoms may emerge as existing ones go away.** For example, if you begin this program with significant joint or muscle aches, as your lymphatic system becomes healthier these pains will go away; however, a healthier lymphatic system may respond to acids by manifesting a discharge of mucus from your nose, which you may call a cold. At its healthiest, no symptoms will be produced by your lymphatic system. However, if you heal your body enough that the pain goes away, but you do not heal it completely, you may be left experiencing more colds than usual. It is like saying that if you start off in California and begin a journey to Nantucket, but stop mid-way, you will remain stuck in a different place (Ohio) unless you complete your journey to its end.

When I was very ill I suffered from daily, excruciating neck pain. When I finally got onto this healing program, this pain became less frequent and less intense, and it eventually disappeared altogether. During the process of its improvement, I experienced a "new" symptom, earaches. Interestingly, I had these often as a child, and never as a teen or adult, when I was extremely unhealthy and ill. These were temporary because I kept on healing my body. I stayed in the car and kept driving down the road. Even though they went away, I could have lived with them had they not. Compared to the neck pain, these were tolerable. This experience was completely positive.

New symptoms that emerge during this process are limited in duration and are never diagnosed as a disease. New healing symptoms may last three days or three months, depending on how "fast you drive." The faster you drive, the faster they will go away.

Your body heals in reverse

Another way to interpret the above concept is to understand that your body heals in reverse. If you have headaches now and ten years ago you had sore throats but no headaches, as your headaches go away, you may experience a very short reoccurrence of your sore throats.

The good and bad news

The good news is that the slower you drive, the less likely you are to experience these new symptoms. Because many of my clients drive too slowly, many of them do not experience these healing reactions. This may be true for many of you, too. The bad news is that the slower you drive, the longer it takes for you to get to the end. So if you do have this experience, view it positively. I always get excited for clients who have these symptoms. I get excited because in 99% of the cases, it means they are aggressively healing their body and will be happy with the quick results.

Correctly Interpreting Your Progress

When you heal you are becoming healthier and new symptoms are not new diseases

When a new symptom erupts in a client, some of them become very worried that they have a new illness. I have helped a number of clients through "false" cancer and other scares, always to find that their fears were unfounded.

If you start out in Ohio and start driving east, you can't get to Utah, where you are less healthy. When you treat symptoms with crutches you are not driving towards health; many times, you are driving towards disease. When you are only treating symptoms with crutches and a new one erupts, it *should* be cause for concern. I understand that this is the experience most people have had, and why they become concerned when something new comes up with this process. If you have not personally experienced this yourself you likely know of someone who has; someone who has been eating "well" and taking vitamins and going to their chiropractor religiously who develops diabetes or cancer, for example. Because people don't realize that they are only treating symptoms, this new condition can be very confusing, scary, and un-empowering. When you understand that you are only treating symptoms with crutches with these other methods and that you are healing with this program, you can better understand the process and feel more certain that any new occurrences in symptoms are most likely due to the healing process.

New diseases and conditions occur when you are *not* healing

A new client contacted me the other day. She has suffered from numerous health problems most of her 50+ years of life. She is currently on a food allergy program and eating a high protein diet. She is feeling much better due to this, but she has had some symptoms that continue undiminished, and she has developed some new ones as well. Her new symptom of rapidly failing eyesight is not due to healing. Another new client came to me eating a similar diet, but with a new diagnosis of an arthritic disease.

Years ago, I worked with another woman who did not like the fact that she could not heal her body "overnight," and after leaving my program she started a high protein diet. About one year later I heard from her again, and this time she had a new diagnosis of diabetes.

High protein diets and other crutches do not heal, and any symptoms that occur while relying on these to look and feel good should be a cause for concern. This is most definitely a sign of the worsening of your health and you should not just wait for it to go away. It won't.

In general, the above examples demonstrate the difference between healing symptoms and symptoms of worsening health. One, if a new symptom occurs while one is eating a high protein diet, or relying on any other crutch, it is almost always the result of a new disease or condition due to deteriorating health. Two, when you heal your body, new symptoms are never labeled as a disease like diabetes or arthritis. And failing eyesight is not a symptom of healing; it is a symptom of degeneration. When you heal your body, you will not experience symptoms of "failing anything."

In all of the above cases, it was the appearance of a new condition that was cause for alarm. It was what motivated the individual to contact me. Of all the many hopes I have for this book, one is that you will get on this healing road before you, too, face greater degeneration in your body. In all three of these particular cases, when the individual presented herself to me she was suffering from an extremely unhealthy bowel and body. While these can be healed, it is much easier to do so prior to it getting to this level.

Healing reactions are temporary

If you are still concerned that a new symptom can be a representation of a new illness, consider this. If it is, your symptom(s) will continue to occur as the months go by, gradually becoming more frequent and more severe. This is the typical pattern of a developing weakness or illness. If your symptoms are due to healing, they will become less frequent and less noticeable as the weeks go by, eventually disappearing.

In the vast majority of cases when a client calls me with a new symptom, as long as it is not an emergency (like a high fever, constant diarrhea, shortness of breath, or excessive bleeding, for example), I make a note of the symptom on their chart and encourage them to keep taking their supplements. I tell them to keep driving the car if they don't like where they are. In most cases, by the time we have our next visit the symptom is gone.

When I work with clients individually I can help them "drive their car" much faster than you who are reading this. Therefore they will get out of Ohio faster than you will; they will see this new symptom go away faster than most of you will.

Watch out for cause and effect conclusions

We are a cause-and-effect society. We have been raised to think this way and it is a very difficult mental and unconscious habit to break. Getting past this is a necessity for you to achieve optimum health and effortless weight maintenance.

We have spent our lives taking aspirin and watching our headaches immediately disappear; eating less or exercising more and watching our weight go down; exerting controlling and threatening behavior on our children and watching them immediately follow our orders without question—all of this without questioning whether or not the long-term effects of these actions are positive and whether or not we are addressing the cause of the problem—the headache, weight gain, or the difficult child, for example.

When we apply an action that yields an immediate positive result we almost assume, *wrongly,* that the action was undeniably correct.

In adopting a cause-and-effect approach to life, we have made some terrible mistakes. Eating a high protein diet and seeing your weight go down is a notorious example of this. Everyone I have ever met who has followed one of these diets believed that they were deficient in protein and that they have lost weight because of their actions to remedy this deficiency. Because the desired weight loss was achieved, it is automatically assumed that the method used to achieve it is correct. On the flip side, when you educate people that their weight problems are a result of poor health and a healthy diet is followed but immediate results are not seen, as it takes time to make your body healthier, this program can be quickly abandoned and labeled as wrong, as the expected cause and effect reaction has not occurred.

When using healing products like *Bowel Strength* and acidophilus, many clients still hold onto this cause-and-effect relationship. Very often I hear comments like, "When I increased the dosage I had more headaches so I reduced it, ", or "When I increased the dosage my bowels were better the next day, or I got the flu, so it had to have been caused by the pills." They are looking for an immediate reaction to changing their dosage, good or bad, because that's how they've been raised to think, yet that's not how this works. **If you continue to look for this cause-and-effect reaction you will get confused and frustrated and quite possibly fail to reach your health and weight goals.**

Bowel Strength and acidophilus are products that help heal your body. Healing takes time. There is no immediate benefit that you will see in taking these; the only immediate reaction that they can cause is loose stools, and even then, many cases of loose stools are due to something other than the Bowel Strength or acidophilus. If you take these pills and the next day fall ill, it is not due to the pills. If you take the pills and feel great the next day, it is not due to the pills. If you take the pills and win the lottery the next day, there is no correlation.

When you use these products and heal your body it is absolutely necessary that you not evaluate your health or your stools on a day-to-day basis. It can take months before there is any noticeable improvement in either. Going too slow and taking too few of the pills is a more common problem, and preventing this is one of my main objectives when working with a client. **Adjusting your supplements according to your symptoms and not according to how your bowel is handling them will almost always guarantee that you heal too slowly.** This way of thinking is very hard to change. It is confusing, but largely because it goes against our inherent desires to see an immediate effect of our actions.

Immediate improvements in your stools can only occur when you use bentonite, as described at the end of this chapter, and immediate improvements in your symptoms, weight, and addictions can only occur when you use the crutches suggested in Chapters 9 and 10.

The fear of feeling bad

While I have repeatedly stated that an excess of *Bowel Strength* or acidophilus can make you feel bad, the occurrence of this is actually quite low. I have to stress it, but it is stressed due to a tendency to treat these products like crutches that treat symptoms; it is not stressed because it is common. It is not.

I understand the fear of feeling bad and of taking something that might make you feel worse. When I was ill, I wrongly blamed a number of products and help I was getting for causing reactions, and then I proceeded to avoid these for many months or years as I convinced myself of their harm.

You don't need to be fearful of these products or this approach. It is the people who are *not* doing this program who should have fear, not you.

If these products are too strong and make you feel bad, you will feel much better one to two days after you stop them. Isn't it worth risking one or two bad days for thousands of good ones? "It is better to have loved and lost than not to have loved at all." It is better to risk a bad day here and there than to not heal your body at all, too. If you do not heal your body, you risk having hundreds of bad days, and an early death, as a result. It is much riskier and much more uncomfortable *not* to heal your body.

Compare apples to apples

As you heal your bowel and body, be sure that you compare apples to apples. I have had clients come to me with poorly formed stools who are following a strict, allergy-free, high protein diet. As they heal their bowel and body, they sometimes find that their stools are still poorly formed, and they can get frustrated with this. When this happens, however, they are comparing apples to oranges. If they have reduced their protein intake and added back wheat and dairy and their stools are poorly formed, then they have made progress. In other words, had they eaten that way when they came to see me on day one, their stools would have been much worse.

Put another way, if you have ten gallons of rain hitting your roof every day and your house gets very wet, and later on you have twenty gallons hitting your roof and your house does not get wetter than it did when only ten gallons hit it, you have made progress! If more rain—from stress, diet, or your environment—hits your roof and you don't feel worse, your roof has gotten stronger.

This can be a sneaky situation. As your body becomes healthier you will likely find that you loosen up the tight controls on your diet that you may have had. This happens gradually and it can be easy to forget "where you used to be."

So, if four months into this program someone says to me they are just as tired as they were before, for example, I might ask, "How much more are you doing and/or eating?" If they are working more, exercising more, and/or eating differently than before, then they have made progress.

Most of your symptoms are not due to healing

Let's say it takes two years or approximately 700 days to heal your bowel and body. If so, there could be about three to five days when the products are too strong, or over 695 days when the supplements are *not* causing your symptoms.

Many of the symptoms that you experience during this process will not be due to the healing process. Understanding the *cause* of your symptoms will help you make the best decision on how to manage them. **Most clients heal their body too slowly and not too quickly. You have a greater risk of feeling bad, or having difficulty losing weight, if you go too slowly than if you go too fast.**

Also, too often people are simply not healing their body and mistakenly assume that all of their health and weight complaints are due to a healing reaction. When I was ill I made the same mistake. I assumed—partly because I wanted to believe at the time that I was actually healing my body—that my neck pain was due to a healing reaction. Two years later, when the pain was no better, I had figured out that it was not a healing reaction causing my problems. This also meant two years of pain and no progress in improving my health.

If you feel worse, you are doing something wrong

We have a "no pain no gain" mentality in this country. It is very wrong to have this mentality when you heal your body. If you feel worse, you will not heal more quickly; you will heal much more slowly, if at all, because it is close to impossible to follow a program when you feel lousy all the time. *When done correctly, this will not be an uncomfortable process.*

Respect your stools!

If you feel worse after eating more fruit, beans, getting Rolfed, a massage, an adjustment, gong therapy or anything else, stop what you are doing. If your stools become more frequent, softer, or looser after one of these, it means that they have caused more acids to go into your bowel than your bowel can handle. When this happens, *the acids get reabsorbed and sent back to where they came from, and in the process, you feel worse because of it.*

Feeling bad or having more frequent or looser stools after a treatment or meal does not mean that you are healing your body and eliminating a lot of acidity; on the contrary. I have seen many people "put up with" these discomforts because they have wrongly been led to believe that while they are suffering, it is helping them. This is sadly not true at all.

Healing reactions are not dangerous

When I was sick I read a book on healing that scared me to death. This was a radical book written many years ago. The author discussed two cases of people who died while attempting to heal their bodies. Their deaths were attributed to the healing process itself, which in this case, was a fast and complete elimination of food for a period of time. The fear these stories created in me lasted for quite a while. All from just one book and two anecdotal stories. Years later, as I learned more about health and healing, I realized that no harm could ever come from it. **On the contrary, millions of people die from not healing their body.**

There is no danger in healing your body unless it is done wrong or you go too slow. When done wrong, you are taking a supplement that is too strong and not respecting this and stopping it as you should. If ten *Bowel Strength* a day gives you diarrhea and you continue taking it anyway, day after day, it could cause harm. However, it means you did not follow the directions I gave you and that most likely, you became impatient and tried to do things your own way.

It can also be dangerous to go too slow. If your body is very unhealthy before starting this program, you may end up with a serious problem if you do not heal fast enough. If you start this program and you are hanging off the edge of a cliff by a string, there may not be enough time to get you up that string and away from the cliff before the wind blows and knocks you into the shark infested waters! If you have 10,000 holes in your roof and you fix one hole a week, you are very vulnerable if a major storm hits, aren't you? It is very rare that I have a client experience this, but it can happen.

One idea for preventing the "going too slow and a dangerous result occurring because of it syndrome" is to be aggressive with this program for at least the first three months. Driving fast may mean a lot of pills initially, but if it saves you—gives you the time to heal—it is worth it. The idea is to drive fast in the beginning so that you get away from that cliff and the possibility of the wind blowing you over it.

If this occurs, call your doctor or go to the hospital

A healing reaction—a positive sign that you are becoming healthier—is not harmful and will not manifest in any of the following ways: frequent diarrhea, difficulty breathing, chest pain, a high fever, excruciating pain, severe dizziness, rapid heartbeat, or large excretions of blood in your urine or stool. If any of these happen get medical attention immediately. These are signs that something is wrong. These do not occur from healing and should never be ignored. Use your common sense. Never put yourself in a place that is potentially dangerous. Better safe than sorry.

Rarely do I have a client experience one of these problems while I am working with them but it can happen. It may happen more likely to you as I cannot, through this book, give you the same aggressive healing advice that I can when I work with someone individually. If your bowel is weak and you are exposed to E-coli, for example, you are likely to become very sick from it. This is best treated medically.

Once I had a client with a heart condition who was on blood thinners and told to use them forever. As her bowel healed, she no longer needed these drugs. They became too strong and this resulted in the frequent urination of blood. This is not a healing reaction. She went to the emergency room and it was discovered that she needed to stop the medications. It could have been very dangerous had she not done so.

If you experience any of the above and it is discovered that your medications are too strong and no longer needed, this is amazing and wonderful news.

Your body is much healthier than it used to be! If one of these above events happens and it is not due to your medication becoming too strong, it means that your body is very weak and vulnerable, and you may want to take this healing stuff more seriously and get more aggressive with it. Sometimes it is the kick that someone needs that they need to heal their body, or go faster in the process.

The elimination of symptoms does not mean you have healed your body

If you have 29 holes in your roof, and the 30th one causes your guest bathroom to get wet when it rains, when you fix this hole the guest bathroom will stay dry, but you still have 29 other holes that cause problems and make your roof—you—less healthy than you could and should be. If your cholesterol recently went up and that goes down early on in this program, for example, this is great, but it does not mean that your entire body is as healthy as it could be. If you keep fixing these holes you will be healthier, and you will also be "further from" your starting point. If you fix 10 holes, it will take much longer to get back to a total of 30 holes, and high cholesterol, than if you only fix one or two of them.

Blood work getting worse

When you heal your body, your blood tests may temporarily worsen. When you heal your bowel, the acids from your organs and fat cells will eventually dump into your bloodstream. Blood tests reflect your body's reactions to these. You have all been falsely led to believe that you are "safe" and healthy if your blood tests come back fine, and so likewise, when these tests are not o.k., you often panic. *The possible temporary worsening of your blood test, and the fear it creates, is one of the challenges you may face when healing your body.*

Pay attention to how you feel. Have you been feeling better, even though this test came out with some items out of range? You are not taking drugs to mask your feelings, and you are not on a high protein diet that does the same, so this feeling better is real. Don't let the blood tests scare you into thinking otherwise.

A good doctor will not overreact to one blood test that is out of range. He will retest this a number of weeks or months down the road. This is important during this process, as the healing of your body will not be consistent, and these blood test results will change.

Many people with cancer and other life-threatening diseases have normal blood work during a time frame very close to their diagnosis. You cannot go from healthy to cancer overnight, so keep in mind that blood tests are misleadingly harmful. It is even more harmful when you are healing your body and this gets interpreted as your health becoming worse, not better, as it actually is.

I have a past client, a fifty-year-old man, who came to me with a diagnosis of liver damage and hepatitis. Throughout the healing process there were times that his liver enzymes spiked, even though he experienced an improvement in his symptoms. As your liver heals—something drugs cannot accomplish— liver enzymes can spike temporarily, as the acids/trash from the "top of your pipe," the stuff that can kill you, moves into the middle of your pipe, "where your liver is," on its way out of your body. If you are really concerned about your blood tests, have a scan done on the organ you are concerned about.

In this case, the client withstood a number of ups and downs in his blood tests, but when his liver biopsy was eventually redone, he was told by the technician that not only was there no more damage, *but that his was the healthiest liver she had ever seen!*

When you are *not* on a healing program, you may experience spikes or imbalances in your blood work. These are to be taken more seriously. When your bloodstream is out of balance, this is because of an excess of acidity in it. This can occur because your organs are healing and dumping acids into it, but it can also happen because an organ is weak and unable to respond properly to buffer the acids in your blood from external sources, like stress and diet.

Is your kitchen a mess because it needs to be remodeled, or is it a mess because you *are* remodeling it?

When you heal your body it is important that you remember that you are becoming healthier, not less healthy. You are driving further away from disease, not closer to it.

Cholesterol tests

Cholesterol tests are the most common blood test results to spike up and down during the healing process. Cholesterol is not regulated by homeostasis, which means that your body will not attempt to correct a level that is too high. When you heal your body, any cholesterol that may be stuck in your arteries, causing them to narrow and putting you at risk of a heart attack, will eventually be sent into your blood to be eliminated. Dr. Dean Ornish is a respected medical doctor who has spent many years devoted to the reversal of heart disease through diet and this worsening of one's cholesterol levels in the blood while the arteries are healing is one he has spent many years documenting. Cholesterol floating in your blood does not kill you. It is the cholesterol that is stuck on your arteries that can. Only a heart scan can measure this for you, and if you are ever concerned about your risk for heart disease, either now or before you begin this program, I strongly advise that you get a scan done. **You are much safer from a heart attack if your heart scan shows no narrowing of your arteries but your blood cholesterol levels are elevated, than if the heart scan shows narrowing of your arteries and your blood cholesterol levels are not elevated.**

In the last fifteen years I have had clients whose blood cholesterol levels have spiked, but I have never had a client die from a heart attack, much less have one.

Have any of you ever remodeled your house? If so, you know that your house can look worse before it looks better. This is true for your blood work as well. *Clients who have infrequent blood tests succeed in this program at a much greater percentage than those who have these done regularly.*

How to Accelerate the Healing Process

The fastest way to heal your bowel is to take an aggressive amount of *Bowel Strength* and/or acidophilus. To heal your body, you need to eliminate your lifetime of accumulated acidity. You could wait for your healthier bowel to do this for you, or you could help your other organs of elimination assist with this process. You will be happier with this process if you help your bowel out.

I consistently find that clients with very unhealthy bowels, who have incorporated the following ideas, are much healthier than those who have not. Some of them "have a lot of holes in their trashcans but a minimum amount of accumulated trash." Typically, the more holes there are in your trashcan, the more trash you will have accumulated in the rest of your house. Usually, the less healthy your bowel is, the less healthy the other organs of your body will be as well. This unhealthy bowel allows for the re-absorption of many more acids that weaken your organs, than a healthy bowel does.

The following suggestions will help you eliminate excess acids that cause health and weight problems. Incorporate as many of these ideas as you can. They will help you look and feel better faster. They do not, however, heal your bowel bacteria nor

227

eliminate the health and weight problems associated with an unhealthy bowel bacterial environment.

Help your other organs eliminate these acids

The majority of acids should be eliminated from your bowel; just like at home, the large trashcan outside holds the majority of my trash that the garbage man clears away every week. But you also have three other, smaller trashcans that can eliminate acids. They are your *kidneys, skin, and lungs*. At home, you have smaller trashcans in the kitchen, bathrooms, etc. to help contain your trash. The more acids that you eliminate through these, the quicker you will heal your body and eliminate the total acidic load in your body. Also, by eliminating some acids through these organs, there will be less that your bowel has to deal with. If your bowel is unhealthy, you will have fewer bowel problems and symptoms if you divert some of the acids out through your other organs of elimination.

Kidney trashcan

To help your kidneys eliminate acids in your urine, drink plenty of pure, uncontaminated water. Distilled or reverse osmosis water is preferable, but spring water is also beneficial. Aim for eight glasses of water per day (64 ounces).

Clients commonly have difficulty drinking this much water every day. Many drink less than three glasses a day. I think the body is the most amazing thing, but there are some flaws. The more water someone needs, and the more dehydrated they are, the less they seem to crave or desire, for example. If this is you, don't worry. You don't have to drink eight glasses of water a day to get healthy. It is simply a helpful way to help heal your body while you are healing your bowel.

As your bowel becomes healthier and better able to eliminate acids, you won't "need" to drink a lot of water to stay hydrated, as your healthy bowel will eliminate the acids that make you vulnerable to dehydration in the first place. Ironically, at this point, you will have a stronger craving/desire to drink water. When I was ill I forced myself to drink almost one gallon, or sixteen glasses of water, a day. I felt better when I did this, but now, with a much healthier body, I drink only about six glasses a day, and I feel thousands of times better than when I drank much more.

Drinking more water will not cause you to retain more; on the contrary. Your body retains water to buffer the un-eliminated acids in your blood. This water comes internally from your tissues. It dehydrates you and this is unhealthy. Drinking more water reduces these acids. It helps your body flush them out through your urine. *The fewer acids that are in your blood, the less water you will retain.*

Numerous studies and claims have been made regarding water consumption— less fatigue, less hunger, less pain, greater mental clarity, and significant reductions in cancer. You may even have come across stories about the "water cure" in which drinking eight glasses a day is said to eliminate numerous health and weight problems. These stories of success indicate that no coffee, tea, chocolate, and alcohol are allowed. So what really helped? Was it the extra water, or the reduction of acidic foods? A person promoting this program told a client that they could have an alcoholic drink, caffeine, or chocolate occasionally after one year of abstinence, but that if these were overdone there would be a set back in symptoms. I would definitely not call this a "cure." You are not cured if you have to constantly depend on something, or avoid something, to help you look or feel better, but drinking water is undoubtedly helpful to your health and will help you feel and look better as you heal your bowel and body.

Skin trashcan

Size-wise, your skin is your largest organ of elimination. To help your body eliminate acids through the pores of your skin, the following are advised: Epsom salt baths, exfoliation, exercise that produces sweat, saunas, and steam rooms.

A hot bath with Epson salts (found at the grocery store or drug store), sea salt, or baking soda added to the bathwater will help draw acids out of your body. Pour one cup into the water and remain in the bath for 20-30 minutes. The water does not have to be hot for these to be of value. In fact, jumping in the salty ocean is just as beneficial. When I was healing my body, I used to get a lot of headaches. While sitting in a hot Epsom salt bath, the headaches would literally go away. Several clients have mentioned that their child's symptoms are greatly improved when they are swimming in the ocean.

Another way to help your body eliminate acids through your skin is with a method called the "blanket sweat." Cover your bed with three or four wool blankets. Take a hot shower, dry off quickly, and wrap your body and head in dry towels. Lie down under the blankets for 15-30 minutes.

Exfoliation helps remove grime and dead skin cells, helping your pores breathe and eliminate better. Using a loofa to scrub your skin while in the shower will also help open your pores and enhance the elimination of acids out of them. When I take a shower, I pour some Epsom salts onto my washcloth and scrub my body with it. If you prefer, you can find some nice, natural exfoliating body scrubs at the health food store and can use those, too. If you have the money, some spas offer a Vichy treatment. During this, your entire body is exfoliated. After your skin is completely rubbed with exfoliates, you are rinsed under a shower while lying on your back. I had a treatment twice and it was heavenly.

It is also important that you don't clog your pores with skin lotions that contain mineral oils. At spas, the products used are specifically chosen because they do not clog pores, a condition most respected for contributing to acne, and termed "comedogenic." Most of the lotions from the drug or grocery store contain mineral oils. Check the label. Instead, choose a lotion made with natural vegetable oils. These do not clog your pores. Most of the lotions in health food stores or spas contain the right oils. Finally, a deodorant is preferable to an antiperspirant, as the latter inhibits the elimination of acidic by-products. If you experience heavy sweating or a strong odor and cannot get away with only using a deodorant, know that as you strengthen your bowel, your sweating and odor will be much less, and one day a deodorant will be all you need.

Far infrared saunas

A home sauna is a luxury that has great value in helping eliminate acids from your body. I am not an expert on saunas, but many of them recommend ones that use far infrared technology.

When I was very ill I used the sauna and steam room all the time. It definitely helped me feel better. I belonged to a gym in Southern California and sometimes I would go simply to use the steam room. I sat in it as long as I could, usually ten minutes or so, then stepped out, drank a lot of water, cooled down a little, and went back in. Afterwards I put on sweatpants and a sweatshirt and drove home with the heat on, even if it wasn't cold, as was often the case.

Sweating problems

As with many body balances, like blood pressure, blood sugar, and body temperature, there is a problem if you sweat too much, but there is also a problem if you don't sweat enough. In a healthy body, strenuous exercise or high temperatures will induce sweating. Many clients who did not "sweat well" initially have found this changed as they healed their bowel and body.

If you have difficulty sweating, any of the above-mentioned suggestions for encouraging this may be stressful and uncomfortable and may need to be avoided until you are healthier.

Lung trashcan

To help eliminate acids through your lungs, learn to breathe deeply, get plenty of fresh air, and avoid toxic chemicals in your environment.

Deep breathing

Every time you exhale, acids are eliminated. When you take shallow breaths, fewer acids are eliminated than when you breathe deeply. When you breathe deeply, your entire belly is moving in and out with your breath, not just your chest. We are born breathing this way. We get into the bad habit of breathing too shallow when we are too busy and don't take the time to relax. Take time every day to focus on your breath, and eventually your habit of breathing shallowly will change. I always focus on my breath when I am lying down to sleep.

Practice deep breathing on your own or join a yoga or Pilates class to help you get used to breathing correctly. Meditate on your own or join a meditation group. A suggested resource is Dr. Weil's Breathing: the Master Key to Self-Healing; www.soundstrue.com; 800-333-9185.

Fresh air and the avoidance of toxic chemicals

Fresh, clean air is wonderful for your lungs. At home, open the windows and turn off the air conditioning as often as possible, if the air outside is clean. For inside your home, consider an air purifier, especially if your house has many odors, irritants like animal fur, or other pollutants. I don't have one, but I don't have any animals, I open my windows to air out my home as often as possible, and I strictly limit the amount of toxic chemicals that I use inside my house.

Awareness about the quality of the air you breathe is helpful. If you paint your room, open the windows. Buy household cleaning products that are non-toxic or make some yourself with ingredients like water and vinegar. If your lungs use up energy and nutrients detoxifying chemicals, less will be available to help them eliminate other toxins, and you will have more health and weight problems because of it.

Rent Another Trashcan While Yours is Being Fixed

In addition to helping your body eliminate acids through your kidney, skin, and lung trashcans, you can also "rent another trashcan." When I remodeled my house I did that, and all of the old kitchen cabinets, flooring, etc was removed much faster because of it. The same is true for your body.

The extra trashcan I recommend to clients is bentonite. Bentonite is clay, and it helps with the absorption of acids in your bowel. It helps your body eliminate the total acid load that has been stored in your body. It helps heal your body. It does nothing to heal your bowel—and a healthy bowel should be eliminating these without the need for bentonite—but until your bowel is healthier, **taking it daily will immediately improve the form and frequency of your bowel movements and as a result, you will lose weight and feel better much faster than if you don't use it.**

To attain your ideal health and weight, two things need to be accomplished: the elimination of old acids, and the healing of your bowel. Bentonite assists with this first one.

Is the bentonite causing symptoms?

If you take bentonite it can trigger a healing reaction, as old acids are quickly moved through your body and into your bowel to be eliminated. The information in this chapter on these reactions is more important to understand if you use it. *While bentonite works very differently from Bowel Strength or acidophilus, a similar concept applies to its use in that if you experience looser stools, very hard and infrequent stools, cramping or any discomfort after taking it, stop it for a few days.*

During the time that you take a break from this, there are only three possible reactions. These reactions, their significance, and how to react to them, are described as follows.

Your stools/bowel movements worsen and/or symptoms do not improve.
This means that the bentonite is not the cause of your symptoms or poor elimination. On the contrary, it was not strong enough to "bind up all of the acids" in your bowel. In this case, your symptoms have flared up because your bowel is weak and it is dealing with an excess of acidity. You cannot fix your bowel right away, but you can try to reduce the acidity that it is struggling with. If your bowels are worse, as defined in Chapter 6, go back to the amount of bentonite that you were taking and reduce the acidic foods that you are eating, rest, drink a lot of water, use the crutches described in Chapter 10,

and try to identify and remove the "rain" that is hitting your roof. Your focus needs to be placed on getting back to your aggressive healing process, because as you reduce the holes in your roof, your house will become less reactive to the rain. As your bowel becomes healthier, you will become less sensitive to these external acids/triggers.

Your stools/bowel movements and/or symptoms remain unchanged. *This means that the bentonite was not causing them.* If your symptoms remain unchanged, follow the directions given previously. Resume the bentonite and focus on reducing the acids in your life.

Your stools/bowel movements and/or symptoms improve. *This means that the bentonite <u>may</u> have been too strong and triggering these problems.* It does not mean for certain that it was. When you are not feeing good, you often automatically slow down your life, rest more, drink more water, and eat better—all of which will help you feel better. If you reduce your bentonite at the same time you do these other things, you may wrongly think it was the reduction that helped you feel better.

In this case, re-try the bentonite in another five days. If your stools worsen and/or the symptoms return within a day or two, it is probably too strong and you should reduce the dosage by half. If you were taking four tablespoons, try two, for example. If you do not have a reoccurrence of your symptoms or your bowels do not worsen one or two days after you re-try it again, it means that they were not the cause of the problem in the first place. In this case, return to the amount you were taking before you stopped it.

Do not start this the same day you start *Bowel Strength* or acidophilus

Because bentonite and *Bowel Strength* and acidophilus can all affect your bowels, do not begin these products at the same time. Start the *Bowel Strength* or acidophilus first, and then after a week or so, when you have found an amount that is not too strong, add in the bentonite and see how your bowel reacts. If your stools are better, great, stay with it. If they get looser, or very slow and hard, reduce or stop it.

You'll need less as you heal

Just as you will eventually need to decrease the amount of *Bowel Strength* or acidophilus that you take, you will eventually need to decrease your bentonite as well. As you eliminate more acids from your body and your body becomes healthier, it will take less bentonite to firm up your stools and help with the elimination of acidity. As time goes by you will need to decrease the dosage, and eventually you will stop it altogether. Pay attention to the frequency and form of elimination, follow the direction above, and you'll get wonderful results with this product.

For more information on bentonite and its use see Chapter 10.

Chapter Nine

The Diet Part is Easy

One reason you are failing to achieve your optimum health and effortless weight maintenance is because you are following diets that are crutches that treat your symptoms, and you not eating diets that are healthy for your body.

On the other hand, eating a healthy diet alone does not mean that you are healthy, and a healthy diet alone will not heal your bowel and body.

In this program, a healthier diet naturally occurs as you heal your bowel and body.

Attempting to manipulate your diet too rapidly will make you less successful with this program, not more. **Your failure to eat "perfectly" will not prevent this program from working.**

Until your bowel and body are healthier, a transition diet is recommended. This includes easy, safe, and healthy dietary crutches, and these are discussed in this chapter.

The Mistaken Power of Diet

Many of you believe that your food choices are much more powerful than they really are. It is common for me to have to explain to a client why all of their healthy eating habits have not somehow miraculously and quickly fixed their health and weight problems. Also, numerous misunderstandings have resulted in great confusion over what you should really be eating, and as a result, a lot of you have been heading down the wrong road. I will explain why there is a large error of understanding in the diet/food area. This understanding will assist you in heading down the right road with your diet, and give you the confidence of knowing that it is the right one.

It takes a long time for a poor diet to harm you

Every time your blood becomes too acidic, *a very gradual weakening* of your organs takes place as un-eliminated acids accumulate. The main sources of acidity are: diet, mental, environmental, chemical, and pharmaceutical stress. If you are thirty-five years old, it has taken thirty-five years of accumulated acidity from *all* of these to create the health and weight problems that you now have. It has taken the combined effects of some 40,000 meals, along with acidity from these other sources, to get you to your current health and weight problems.

Therefore, if you begin eating a healthier diet, it is absolutely unreasonable to expect even one year's worth of better eating--some 1000 meals-- to have the power to offset the harm done by 40,000 meals, mental, environmental, and other stressors, not to mention the unhealthy bowel you inherited when you were born!

Eating healthy does not mean that *you* are healthy!

When you starve yourself, exercise ferociously, or eat a high protein diet, you *force* your body to convert fat deposits into glucose (energy), thereby losing weight. Every day your body needs a certain amount of glucose, so on any day that this is inefficient, fat and weight will drop off. High protein diets keep the acids out of your blood, which results in a reduction of symptoms and much less water weight as well. You are used to losing weight and/or feeling better immediately on these programs.

When you diet, you lose weight right away, and so when you eat healthier, you expect to *be* healthier right away too. You have been led to believe that you can change your health and weight conditions overnight, and this is a wrong and harmful mentality to have.

The process of fat conversion into glucose, for example, is entirely different from the process of healing your body. In the first case, you have taken your broken car and attached it to a tow hook and are able to reach your destination. In the second case, you have spent time repairing your car, only after which you can set off for your destination. In the first case you get results faster, but your car still doesn't work, and you must use a tow all your life-- i.e., starve yourself or eat a dangerous high protein diet all your life to keep the weight off. In the second case, you arrive at your destination (low weight) after a longer period of time, but once there, you remain there effortlessly and easily.

Put another way, just because you arrive at your destination does not mean that your car is working. Just because you lose weight does not mean that your body is working. When you lose weight quickly, your body is definitely not working better. **When you lose weight or feel better overnight you have not become healthier overnight as well. Just because you are thin or symptom free, does not mean that you are healthy.**

You cannot quickly heal your bowel and body with a change in your diet. There are no "magical diets." You may lose some weight, but your body cannot quickly become healthier in the process, and it is a healthy body that will keep the weight off and keep you cancer free, too.

If it sounds too good to be true, it is (not true!)

Any diet that works "magic" will fail you. I just read about the billions of dollars of money lost by investors who fell for a Ponzi scheme run by an affluent businessman. Many people have had their lives completely destroyed as a result and believing that high returns on their investment were legitimate. This financial investment sounded too good to be true, and it was! It takes hard work and commitment to make a lot of money, and it takes hard work and commitment to make your body healthier, too.

If a food immediately helps you lose weight or feel better, it does not mean that food is healthy

There is a strong and popular tendency to judge the health of a food based upon its immediate effect on your weight and symptoms. If you eat a certain way and lose weight, you tend to conclude that it is a healthy diet. If you eat a certain way and feel better right away, the same conclusion is drawn. This approach is wrong and leads to continual health and weight struggles in the long-term.

When I was very unhealthy I felt better when I was drinking and doing drugs, but that doesn't mean they were good for me. This improvement in how you feel is the primary reason you become so addicted to these behaviors. Likewise, many people feel bad after eating whole wheat bread, but that is not because whole wheat bread is bad for you.

Some foods are healthy for you that can, in the short-term, make you feel bad or gain weight.

Some foods are not healthy for you that can, in the short-term, make you feel good and lose weight.

237

How does this happen? If your bowel is unhealthy and you try to eat a healthy, high fiber diet, you will have a hard time breaking down the fiber. This will make you gassy, bloated, and uncomfortable. The reason this way of eating causes this discomfort is not because high fiber foods are bad for you, it is because your bowel is unhealthy. If your bowel is unhealthy and unable to efficiently eliminate acids, eating a high carbohydrate diet will cause you to retain water and your weight will go up. This type of diet is not bad for you either and is not the cause of your weight gain. An unhealthy bowel causes your weight gain.

If a high carbohydrate diet makes you look and feel bad and you respond by eating a high protein diet, your bowel will become less healthy. This will make it even more difficult to lose weight in the future. This is a current reality. *Because your bowels are unhealthy and you are eating for how you feel and not for how healthy the diet is, you are eating an unhealthy diet, and the vicious cycle of eating poorly, making your organs less healthy, and then finding it more uncomfortable to eat healthfully and lose weight and feel better in the future has developed.*

It is much easier to learn about quick fixes than it is to learn how to use diet to heal

Many people have read about and/or tried one variation or another of food avoidance, which often falls under the heading of food allergies or intolerances. There are many health and weight loss books on the market that rely on this approach, and the majority of my peers utilize this method in their practices as well.

If your roof has holes in it you will feel better immediately if you avoid rain, or the foods that irritate it. You can quickly erect a structure over your roof and protect it from the rain, but because your house doesn't get wet does not mean that it is stronger. This is the deception of these allergy diets. Because people feel better right away, they are misled into thinking that they got healthier right away, too. **To become healthier you must "fix the holes in your roof," as this program does, and this takes time.**

In part, it is because of the ease in learning and teaching this food allergy approach that it is widely used. It does not even take an education to do this. Plenty of information on food allergy and avoidance diets can be found in books and online. You do not need a practitioner to provide this for you.

Learning how to heal your body is entirely different. I could put a tarp on my roof at home, but I could not build a new house. And building a new body is thousands of times more complex than building a new house. I have spent thousands of hours learning this process.

You shouldn't have to eat perfectly to look and feel good—I don't!

When I was ill I changed my diet drastically and felt a little better. As soon as I wondered off of this extremely strict diet, I was debilitated. Today, I can eat poorly and not feel bad. Following a very strict diet was stressful and it made me feel like a social outcast, and I do not believe that it was beneficial to my health to be eating "perfectly" but feeling emotionally stressed. Also, I was long deceived into thinking that I was healthier than I was just because I could manipulate my symptoms with my diet.

A strong roof can tolerate some heavy rainstorms without incurring damage. A strong roof will also prevent the rain from leaking into your house. When your body is healthy, it too will be able to tolerate any food that it is given—whether it is sugar, wheat, dairy, citrus fruits—you name it. **If you have to avoid any food to look and feel better, your body is not as healthy as it could be.**

Since healing my body, I crave healthy foods. I eat these most of the time. But I also eat less healthy foods at times, because it is easier to function socially without following a strict diet. For many years I had to avoid a lot of foods to prevent myself from feeling horrible, and I now also enjoy the power of knowing that I can be flexible and much less controlling with my diet.

The Ultimate Guide for Unraveling Dietary Confusion

For every one of you who are desperately trying to improve your health but are completely frustrated with all of the conflicting advice, I understand. When I was extremely ill, I was willing to do whatever it took to get better. I made extreme and radical changes in my diet. I forced myself to eat many foods that I was told I needed to eat, in the hopes of getting better. One practitioner told me I had to eat alfalfa sprouts every day. I hated these. I would put in a mouthful and chase them down with a huge glass of water. I went from a pre-illness diet of refined carbohydrates, steak, and sugar to a diet of millet, quinoa, brown rice, vegetables, fish, liver, and yogurt. Except for the fish, these were all foods I had never eaten before. Most of them I had never even heard of before, like kohlrabi, sun chokes, amasake, and essene bread.

I tried numerous dietary programs for a long time without improvement. During this time, I began my own quest for answers and voraciously read all of the books I could on diet, health, and healing. Even twenty years ago, the dietary advice was conflicting, yet it was always presented with the strong conviction that "their way" was the answer. I was very ill and I got that I couldn't afford to make the wrong choice for too long, but how could I know which was the right one? I understand how most cancer patients feel when I see them. Understandably, they are especially overwhelmed with the contradictions and fear of choosing the wrong path.

I will help you eliminate these dietary frustrations and confusion. Having gotten to where I am today, the ability to unravel these is very comforting. I feel very lucky to be here.

How do you know if what I have to say about diet is right?

The dietary advice in this book is based on science and physiology, but even science can be twisted and manipulated to serve anyone's purpose! The advice in this book is based on common sense, but let's face it, sometimes you don't have much of this, especially when you are scared or uncomfortable. It is also based on over sixteen years of experience helping clients, but then again, I know plenty of practitioners who have worked twice as long as I have who are dispensing dangerous dietary advice. It is based on the fact that long-term studies support it; unfortunately, given the cost of such studies, not many have been done, and you can find many short-term ones to contradict it. So how do you judge whether this advice is right?

Ultimately, the beauty of this program is that you don't have to worry about the right way to eat. It will happen naturally.

Still, does it make sense?

Twenty-three countries have a life expectancy greater than ours, even though they use fewer medications and sophisticated surgeries to keep them alive. We can, and have, learned a lot about health by looking at the lifestyles of people in these other countries. For example, the Asians have eaten a low protein diet for thousands of years. In the United States, one would be led to believe that this contributes to obesity, arthritis, migraines, and on and on. On the contrary, the Asian population is much thinner than we are and suffer less illness overall.

When I first became ill I was given a lot of conflicting dietary advice. Before I was educated enough to know better, I often thought about the health of other countries and their traditional diets, and if the information that I was given conflicted with what I had learned about them, I'd be leery of following it. For example, I was told that eating carbohydrates feeds yeast and that I had a major yeast overgrowth in my body. The solution was to greatly reduce my carbohydrate load. I did this for a while and temporarily felt a little better, only to feel worse later. At some point, I thought, wait a minute, if a high-carbohydrate diet feeds yeast, then the Asians must be crammed full of it and its related problems, but they're not, so that doesn't make much sense. As you learn more about nutrition, physiology, and biochemistry, looking overseas may prove valuable to you as well. At the very least, it's a place to begin, and to start asking questions. Thinking through some of the nutritional advice you receive may save you a lot of money, time, and effort down the road. It may save your life as well.

A Healthy Body Will Crave and Tolerate a Healthy Diet

Ultimately, this is the answer to your confusion. A healthy body can eat a lot of carbohydrates, fiber, cheese, gluten, and spicy foods and look and feel great doing so. A healthy body feels good even when rain is hitting its roof. A healthy body craves grains and vegetables, and finds meat proteins and sugar unappealing.

When you heal your bowel and body, you will eat food as nourishment. Less will be needed and desired. You will have no cravings. I used to love alcohol and sugar. I couldn't resist them. I can now, effortlessly (which still completely amazes me.) A healthy body rejects these stimulants. Also, it used to be that if someone asked me where or what I wanted for dinner, I had a strong opinion based on what I was craving. Now, it never matters. I never care where we go out to eat, for example. I can make do anywhere.

Today I eat a largely vegetarian diet. This is what I love and crave. But, don't read this and think to yourself, forget it, I couldn't eat that way. I'm not doing this. You do not need to be a vegetarian for this to work. In fact, I don't want you to give up animal protein right away. You will feel worse if you do and will be more likely to quit the program. Heal your body and see where it takes you. **My clients naturally, easily, and effortlessly give up meat proteins, coffee, sugar, alcohol and other unhealthy substances as they heal their**

bowel and body. It is an end result, not an immediate direction to be taken at the beginning of this journey.

Fear of the dietician

When I first became ill I went to many conventional doctors. Early on in this process, I also considered seeing a dietician (I had never heard of someone called a nutritionist), because I knew my diet was horrendous and it made sense that it was contributing to my illness. But I was afraid to go. I was afraid that she would tell me what I already knew; that I needed to eat more fruits and vegetables and less sugar. I didn't need someone to tell me this. And I didn't know how I could follow this advice because I didn't like eating very many fruits or vegetables, and I craved sugar. I was embarrassed to tell someone how poorly I ate and feared being reprimanded for it. So I didn't go.

The fear of changing one's diet is very common. I believe that it is the number one reason someone will not seek help with healing his or her body. I understand. But I also want to scream out loud, "You don't need to worry. The diet part of this is actually extremely easy. When you heal your bowel, your body chemistry will change, and you will like and crave foods that you never imagined you would. You will dislike unhealthy foods that you never thought you would be able to give up."

Increased sensitivity to unhealthy foods

In addition to craving less animal protein, sugar, coffee, and other highly acidic foods and beverages, you may also find that during this process you are more sensitive to these foods. Sometimes a client enters my office that likes and drinks coffee daily. This habit provides pleasure and no discomforts. As their body becomes healthier, they usually find that after they drink coffee, they don't feel good anymore. They may feel jittery, or it may cause their stools to become loose, even though this never used to happen.

As your body becomes healthier, it does a better job of "moving acidity" from your blood into your organs of elimination. Your liver becomes healthier before your bowel, for example, and this can mean that all of a sudden, when you drink alcohol, it is quickly metabolized and the acids of it are sent into your bowel, causing loose stools, because your bowel is not completely healed yet. If your liver is weak, you can drink alcohol and, in this case, the acids from it do not find their way into your bowel. Instead, they may simply kill off a liver cell. In the long run, this is very dangerous for you, but in the short-term, it does not produce discomforts like loose stools. You can dangerously believe that the alcohol is not hurting you. When you heal, the true health of a food will be revealed. Highly acidic foods and drinks will produce discomfort when you have them, and while this can be initially confusing, it is a great blessing. **A healthy body will reject unhealthy foods and beverages.**

The physical reaction to food and beverages precedes the emotional one and an inevitable discontinuance of them. If a client has been drinking coffee for a long time, they have developed a physical *and* emotional attachment to it. When their body becomes healthier and physically reacts to it in a negative way, it takes a little longer for their brain to catch up. They have developed years of unconscious associations between the coffee and pleasure gained in drinking it. It takes a little time to switch this around. Typically this person will find that their body no longer desires it but their brain does. After a little while, however, their brain develops new associations with the coffee—unpleasant ones—that ultimately make it effortless to stop this habit.

Focus on your bowel and the diet will come

This program is not about eating whatever you want and becoming thin and healthy. All of the diets and other programs that make these claims should be avoided and eyed very suspiciously. If it sounds too good to be true, it almost always is!

You don't need to eat great to heal your bowel and body. You *will* eat great at the end of the program because you will crave healthy foods and you will not crave unhealthy ones. Trust and patience, you need these. Don't force a change. You will fail if you do. Let your body get healthier and your blood chemistry to become more balanced, and your cravings will change. Ninety percent of what I crave and love to eat today are foods that I never would have eaten twenty years ago.

Follow this program and see what happens to your diet. I am certain that you will know it is not only right when you get to it, but that deep down, you will feel more confident about your long- term health eating this way. You will get it that when you wanted and felt and looked better eating animal protein, you were not healthy, for example.

In the end you will find that you are eating to survive, not for the thrill. Your thrills will come from feeling and looking great, feeling in control, and being fearless of disease. I've been on both roller coasters, and this one is 100% better.

You will feel worse and quit healing your body if you eat perfectly now

A "perfect" diet is low in protein, but until your bowel is healthier, this diet will make you look and feel worse. Until your bowel is healthier, you will not be able to eliminate all dietary crutches, like alcohol, sugar, and large amounts of protein, and feel good doing so. If you try you will fail, and feeling like a failure is both unnecessary and unproductive. You will be *discouraged*, not encouraged, to continue with this healing program. If you make severe sacrifices to eat perfectly you will have high expectations. You will expect your bowel and body to heal quickly given your sacrifices, and you will be very discouraged when this does not happen. It cannot happen. It will backfire on you.

A perfectly healthy diet is not needed to heal your bowel and body. Once these are healed, a healthy diet will be effortless to maintain.

The top of the mountain

It is very hard for my clients to believe and trust that one day they will no longer desire their food addictions—whether it is coffee, sugar, alcohol, or meats. They have a hard time believing that they will be able to eat gluten one day, when they are very intolerant of it now. When it occurs, the effect is very powerful. At this point, these clients are very easy to help. This effect gives them great faith in this program and in their body. This is usually a new experience, and a profound one, at that. I call this point the "top of the mountain." While this is not the finish line, running down the mountain is much easier than running up it, and the empowerment that comes from this experience puts them at the top.

The other day a client, who has dieted and lost and regained weight many times, told me that she was getting rid of her fat clothes, because this time, she knew she was never going to need them again. Her fear of regaining weight was gone, for the first time ever!

Food allergies and intolerances

An unhealthy bowel causes food allergies and intolerances. If you have food allergies or find that some foods cause discomfort, leave these out of your diet until your bowel and body are healed. Later on, after you have spent time healing your bowel and have noticed improvements in it, try a food that once was problematic. Do this with foods that caused discomfort but not with foods that triggered life-threatening allergic reactions. Work with your allergist and wait until your allergy test shows that you are no longer allergic to them before adding these into your diet. Because almost everyone else is treating symptoms with crutches, and this approach means that you will likely be "allergic forever," your allergist will be skeptical that you can eliminate your food allergies (or maybe you will be told that you will outgrow them, only to "grow into" a worse health problem later on). It may be up to you to request that a test be re-done.

The Qualities of a Food or Beverage That Make it Healthy For You

Popular dietary advice puts too much focus on nutritional, protein, fat, and/or caloric content and not on the healing ability of a food. A food that is low in fat and calories can be very unhealthy for you, and vice versa. The continued focus on these variables is one reason you have been led astray, confused, frustrated, and in many cases, given up.

A healthy body will be a thin, symptom-free, addiction-free, disease-free one. The three most important variables to consider in determining if a food is *healthy* for you are: its digestibility, pH value, and nutrient content.

Digestibility is important because when a food is difficult to digest, a lot of energy goes towards the digestion of it, leaving less energy available to heal your body and eliminate acids. The workmen cannot be remodeling your house and sitting down to a big lunch at the same time. Additionally, poorly digested foods create additional acids, and this means greater weakness in your body and more health and weight problems.

The **pH value** is important because if you eat foods that are too acidic or too alkaline, excess stress is placed on your body to correct this imbalance and increased damage and ill health occurs. In particular, a high-acid diet, like the very popular reduced carbohydrate diet, makes your bowel and body less healthy. The goal in this program is to eliminate the acids that cause health and weight problems, not add to them.

The **nutrient content** is important because your body uses vitamins and minerals from food to build new cells/organs. Often too much focus is placed on a foods nutrient content with disregard to its pH and/or digestibility. Putting vegetables into sugar-laden products is wrong. Commending steak for its iron content when it is highly acidic and very difficult to digest is misleading and wrong too. The entire picture needs to be considered.

It is particularly important that you understand the importance of digestibility, pH and nutrient content if you have been led to believe that exercise is "everything;" that as long as you exercise regularly you will prevent health and weight problems from occurring. Exercise is very beneficial, however if you exercise and do not concurrently eat healthy foods, as defined above, you *will* end up with health conditions and premature disease and death.

In summary, your body needs nutrients to build new, healthy organs (nutrient content), it needs the time to do this (digestibility), and it cannot progress forward if it is constantly being torn apart (pH value).

If you choose low acid, easy to digest foods, your diet will automatically be nutritious. For this reason, the following information will focus on the digestibility and pH value of foods only.

Dietary Changes/Crutches to Use *Now*

Although you will crave a healthier diet as your bowel and body heals, I suggest you incorporate some easy diet changes now. These can help you look and feel better now, while you are waiting for your bowel and body to become healthier. A healthier diet will also reduce, but not eliminate, some of the crutches recommended in Chapter 10.

Replace high acid foods with similar high alkaline ones

Highly acidic foods are unhealthy and in the short-term, they can make you look and feel bad; highly alkaline ones are healthy and in the short-term, they can help you look and feel better by buffering the un-eliminated acids in your blood.

Sugar, distilled and wine vinegar, salt, coffee, soda, and hydrogenated fats are highly acidic. Replace these with similar items that are alkalinizing. For example, use honey and maple syrup to replace sugar and sucrose; grain, balsamic, apple cider and rice vinegar to replace distilled and wine vinegar; sea salt to replace salt; black tea to replace coffee; and olive oil and expeller-pressed vegetable oils to replace hydrogenated fats. Carbonated drinks are highly acidic, even carbonated water. Stay away from these now. Spend a few minutes looking at your food labels and avoid these highly acidic ingredients as much as possible. Many products that use these similar, but alkaline and therefore healthy, ingredients can be found in the health food aisle of your grocery store or in your local health food store.

And choose less acidic foods

Eggs are less acidic when cooked lightly and the egg yolk is still soft. Milk is highly acidic, but dairy products like yogurt and cheese are much less so due to the added enzymes that helps with their digestion.

Eat high quality foods, if you can afford to. A high quality wine is less acidic than a cheap one. High quality, organic beef is less acidic than cheaper cuts of meat, etc.

Minimize processed cheese food, like American cheese. Eat the real thing. Cheddar, Swiss, Brie, mozzarella, etc are low acid, easy to digest foods. If you have a dairy allergy or intolerance, wait to introduce these until your bowel and body are healthier.

Try to replace cow's milk, even low and non-fat, with rice or soymilk. I'm a fan of rice milk. Don't knock it until you've tried it. You might not want to sit down and drink a glass of it, but on cereal, in a smoothie, or in mashed potatoes, for example, few of you will notice a difference. Do you like white rice? If you do, you will most likely enjoy rice milk as well. Try a non-dairy ice cream. There are a number of decent tasting ones made from soy and rice milk. Yogurt is also easier to digest, and less acidic, than cow's milk. (Young babies and children need more protein and calcium than rice or soy can provide. It is best to give them yogurt and cheese in place of cow's milk as much as possible due to the high incidence of dairy allergies and problems associated with eating it.)

Better protein foods for now

It takes some time to heal your bowel and change an environment that is host to 100 trillion bacteria. While you are healing it, you will look and feel better if you keep your protein intake higher than is ideal. This slows down the movement of acids into your blood and bowel.

On the other hand, high protein foods are very acidic and damaging to your bowel and body. You can help the healing process by eating proteins that are lower in acidity and easier to digest. *Replace as much of the beef, pork, turkey, and chicken that you eat with fish (except shellfish like lobster and crab), eggs (especially soft-cooked ones), tofu, cottage cheese, yogurt, and rice, whey and soy protein powders.*

I have one important warning for you, however. These foods are high in protein, yet except for fish, they do not have as much protein as chicken, turkey, and meats. If you replace all of the chicken and meat you eat with these foods you can still experience some discomfort or weight gain as a result. If you make this switch, consider that four eggs or two to four scoops of protein powder would need to be eaten to replace approximately a tiny three or four ounces of chicken or meat. So proceed slowly, and if your bowel movements become more frequent and/or looser, or if you experience any discomfort or weight gain, go back to your higher protein diet and try this again later on, when your bowel is healthier and better able to handle the release of acids that accompanies a lower protein diet.

Likewise, soy does not cause disease and any claims that it does are the result of the misunderstanding that lower protein foods cause your body to cleanse and this causes problems when your bowel is too unhealthy to eliminate these acids. Soy is lower in protein than chicken, beef, etc., so if you switch to soy products. Therefore, when people switch to soy products and reduce their other high protein foods, the ill effects of this switch are due to their unhealthy bowels, not to the soy itself!

Don't force changes

Let your healthier bowel and body tell you when it is ready to eat a healthier, lower protein diet. Waiting for your body to reject a higher protein diet is very different from forcing this to happen. Do not try to control this. Let it happen and trust that it will. When you allow this to happen, the switch to a lower protein diet will be very comfortable and effortless.

Dietary Help for Your Bowel

The fastest way to heal your bowel is to use an aggressive, individualized dose of *Bowel Strength* or acidophilus. The following dietary suggestions also help; however do not expect them to heal it much more quickly. **It takes a very long time for dietary and other acids to weaken your bowel. You cannot reverse this quickly simply by eating healthier.**

I present this information, however, because clients have wrongly been told to avoid some of these healing foods, and because you have to eat something, so why not try to make it something that helps you achieve your health and weight goals.

The alkalinizing diet suggestions presented earlier will also help heal your bowel, as they help create a pH in your bowel that is necessary for your good bacteria to grow. An alkaline diet also reduces the total acid load in your body and reduces the amount of "trash" that has to be eliminated. An easy-to-digest diet helps because it helps your body eliminate acids more efficiently, and excess acids weaken all of your organs, including your bowel.

In the short-term, the inclusion of some highly alkaline foods will help you heal your bowel and body faster. They will also help you feel better faster. However, just as it is important to eventually stop the *Bowel Strength* or acidophilus, it is likewise important that, one day, you move away from these highly alkaline foods. The ideal pH of your blood is neither too alkaline nor too acidic, and a long-term diet is neither too alkaline nor too acidic, either.

While you are healing your bowel, the following foods and beverages are helpful to the healing process. They will also help you feel better in the short-term. This includes: lemons and lime and their juices, grapefruit and grapefruit juice, garlic, and onions.

On the other hand, limit the following "healthy, high alkaline foods" until your bowel is healthier, as they can exacerbate your health and weight problems: Oranges and orange juice, grape juice, tomato juice, raisins, and spicy peppers like jalapenos, chili, and curry.

Not all citrus is created equally. Grapefruit and orange juice affect your bowel differently. Citrus fruit is very alkalinizing, not acidic, as is commonly thought. It is also very cleansing, and can either be valuable, or trigger discomforts, depending on the health of your bowel. When your bowel is unhealthy, grapefruit is healing to it. Sadly, people with unhealthy bowels have often been told to avoid *all* citrus, which means that they have been avoiding foods—grapefruit, lemons, and limes—that could have been helping heal their bowel. (By the way, as reported in *Alternative Medicine* magazine, September 2005, a study in Chicago at the Smell & Taste Treatment and Research Foundation found that when men smell the aroma of a grapefruit they perceived women to be six years younger than their actual age!)

Some medications should not to be taken with grapefruit, so consult with your doctor if you are taking medications before incorporating grapefruit into your diet.

Probiotic and prebiotic foods

Probiotics contain beneficial bacteria and directly help improve the status of yours. Foods that contain probiotics include yogurt, kefir, miso, tempeh, and sauerkraut. *While these are healthy for your bowel, they cannot replace the Bowel Strength and/or acidophilus.* They would never be strong enough to heal your bowel all on their own.

Likewise, the now popular kombucha tea is great too, but do not use this to heal your bowel either. Like yogurt, kefir, and miso, the amount of cultures in this beverage is completely insignificant to heal your bowel. The above drinks and foods are easy to digest, low in acidity or alkalinizing, and they fit the description of foods that help create and maintain health. The small amount of cultures in them also make them good for maintaining, *but not fixing*, a healthy bowel. As always, if you have a dairy allergy, avoid yogurt and kefir until your allergy is gone.

Kombucha tea is alkalinizing and for this reason, it can help you immediately feel and look a little better. Also, the caffeine and sugar provide you with immediate energy, and everyone feels better with more energy. To conclude, however, that this drink has immediately healed your bowel is wrong. This does not happen. The immediate benefit is from the two items I mentioned above, and too many people have wrongly concluded that their bowel was healed "overnight" because they felt better overnight.

Prebiotics are indigestible ingredients that stimulate the growth of the beneficial bacteria in your bowel by providing nutrients they need to survive and multiply. Foods that contain prebiotics include whole grains, legumes, many vegetables and fruits, including onions, dark green leafy vegetables, asparagus, artichokes, bananas, garlic, leeks, berries and bananas, lemons and limes, flaxseed, oats, apples, grapefruit, barley, foods containing inulin, including some yogurts and non-dairy frozen deserts, and fructo-oligosaccharides (FOS). Prebiotics have also been found to reduce intestinal problems like constipation, Chrohn's disease and inflammatory bowel disease, lower cholesterol, prevent colorectal cancer, enhance the immune system, and improve your body's uptake of calcium.

The allium family--which includes garlic, onions, leeks, shallots, scallions and chives-- has been shown to destroy harmful bacteria in your bowel. Garlic can eradicate thirty different types of harmful bacteria and fungi, as well as inhibit gastrointestinal ulcers and many types of low-grade infections. Additionally, it has been found that people who consume lots of garlic and onions show reduced rates of cancers of the skin, stomach, liver, colon, lungs, and cervix. The sulfur compounds in onions help lower dangerous levels of blood fats and keep plaque from adhering to your artery walls. Garlic contains natural anticoagulants that help thin your blood and protect against platelet stickiness, thus lowering the risk of clotting and stroke.

Lamb intestines!

When I read my all-time favorite book, "Eat, Pray, and Love," the author described eating a dish of lamb intestines in Rome. This doesn't sound too good to me, but I bet it is great for your bowel. As much as I would love to travel all over the world for pleasure, my greatest interest in this is to observe the traditional diets of much healthier, thinner countries, particularly in regard to the qualities that help make it healthy for the bowel. Sauerkraut in Germany and miso soup in Japan are two more examples of traditional foods consumed elsewhere that are healing to your bowel. Most traditional American foods don't have these qualities, such as hamburgers, fries, soda, pizza, and fried chicken. These do nothing but weaken your bowel!

B.R.A.T. Diet: <u>B</u>ananas, <u>R</u>ice (white), <u>A</u>pples, <u>T</u>ea (black)

I first learned about this diet from the medical profession over twenty years ago. Since then, this safe and effective method for reducing loose stools seems to have been completely forgotten and replaced with the "easier" drug-taking movement. While it is easier to use drugs to treat diarrhea, it is not safe in the long run and will eventually contribute to a less healthy bowel; it will make the cause of the problem worse in the long run.

If you experience diarrhea, stop all food except the above for a day. One day should suffice for firming up your stools. If not, continue eating these foods another day, but again, see your doctor if the diarrhea persists more than two days, becomes more than four times a day, or is accompanied by a fever, difficulty breathing, or any other symptoms that are debilitating or potentially dangerous.

Apples and apple juice affect your body and bowel differently. For firming up your stools, make sure that you eat only whole apples or applesauce. Apples can be eaten raw, but are best without the skin if your stools are loose. Filtered apple juice has had the pectin removed, the ingredient that helps bind up the acids in your bowel and firm up the stool. Unfiltered apple juice has a little more pectin in it, but still not enough to be helpful. In fact, drinking apple juice can make your stools looser, not firmer.

Eat as many bananas as you can when your stools are loose, and do not worry that this will make you fat; on the contrary, well-formed stools help with the elimination of acids that cause water weight and fat production, and bananas support this. White rice won't make you fat, either.

Black tea is especially helpful for firming up your stools. Black tea contains tannins that have been proven to help bind the contents of your bowel. If you have diarrhea, drink your tea plain or sweetened with honey.

If your stools are not loose, these foods are still valuable in helping your body eliminate acids from your bowel and body and can help you look and feel better while you heal. Eat them as often as you can.

Stop stressing out about white rice

Every time I advise a client to eat a lot of white rice they freak out. I think this is because many people have heard that white flour products are horrible and cause weight gain and illness, and they have lumped white rice in with these products. *White rice and white flour are not the same.*

Rice is a carbohydrate—of which a healthy body needs a lot—but it is easier to digest and less acidic than the refined wheat products that make up the majority of carbohydrates that Americans consume. Unfortunately, all of this refined wheat has given carbohydrates a bad name. There is a significant difference between how your body handles rice and how it handles refined wheat products.

White rice is much easier to digest and much less acidic than white flour. White rice is very soothing to your bowel; white flour is very irritating. White flour products can make your stools looser and worse; white rice has the opposite effect. Firmer stools result in fewer symptoms, better health, and a healthier weight.

White rice cereal is the first solid food, after pureed fruits and vegetables that we are told to feed our babies. Do you know why? The reason is that rice is very easy to digest. Are we told to feed our babies bagels or chicken at five months? No. Do you know of any one who is allergic to white rice? I don't. This is another reason it is a wonderful food to eat.

If you are still uncertain about this suggestion, think about the Asian countries that have been consuming white rice as a staple part of their diet for thousands of years. They are thinner and healthier than we are, and they have survived on this diet for thousands of years. Personally, I don't think that America is going to survive on our diet and the diet advice we have been following for three hundred years, much less three thousand, like the white-rice eating Asians!

White rice has less fiber than brown, which is a benefit to those of you with an unhealthy intestinal bacterial environment that cannot digest fiber comfortably. In this case, eating white over brown is a better choice as it reduces the gas and bloating some experience after eating brown rice.

Replace as many of your other carbohydrates with white rice as possible. Eat less bread and pasta and more white rice, for example. **Do not replace your protein foods with white rice until your bowel is healthier.**

Unfortunately, many American food restaurants don't serve rice, and many Chinese restaurants that do serve it, use unhealthy processed soy sauce on their dishes. If there are enough requests, maybe more restaurants will serve rice. In the meantime, you can easily cook it yourself. I make a pot and store the remainder in the refrigerator and then simply reheat it when needed. Cooked rice will keep in the refrigerator for about four days. Stay away from the highly processed varieties of white rice, like minute-rice, and instead try white basmati or jasmine rice. Some quick ideas for toppings are: sautéed vegetables in olive oil and garlic; salsa; butter and parmesan cheese; soy milk and cinnamon; soy sauce that is made with sea salt ("Eden" foods makes one); lemon juice, parsley, and butter; butter and sliced almonds; melted butter, chopped cilantro, and avocado slices; olive oil, butter, and sesame seeds; pesto; and cayenne pepper, olive oil, and roasted pumpkin seeds. (Butter is also easy to digest and low in acidity. It is not the cause of your health and weight problems.)

Reduce high fiber foods for *now*

When vegetables are raw, or uncooked, they contain more fiber than when they are cooked, because heat breaks down the fiber in food. Salads, beans, nuts, bran, and even cooked broccoli, cauliflower, and broccoli are high in fiber and are best for people who have a strong bacterial environment in their bowel, as this prevents gas, bloating, looser stools, and other discomforts after eating these. My clients find that they tolerate, enjoy, and crave a higher fiber diet when their bowel becomes healthier.

The more sour the better

Sourdough is an easy to digest carbohydrate and as long as you are not allergic to gluten, it is excellent to eat this while you are healing your bowel bacteria. The more sour the bread, the better it is for you. San Francisco sourdough is my favorite, but since that it hard to find where I live, I purchase sourdough from one of the local bread shops. I can even get amazing sourdough pancakes at a local restaurant. If you travel to Europe you will find soured bread all over the place. I've worked with a number of clients who try to avoid bread for their weight but eat a large quantity of it when they are in Europe and end up losing, not gaining, weight while doing so. My kids prefer sourdough bread to whole wheat.

A Summary of Good Foods to Eat Now

To simplify the above information, the following is a list of foods and beverages that are great to eat now, while you are healing your bowel and body, to help you look and feel better. I am in no way implying that these are the only foods you should eat; rather, I am suggesting that you eat more of them than you currently do and that the more you have, the better you will look and feel. Once you have healed your bowel and body these ideas are still good to maintain in your daily or weekly diet. This list includes:

Fruit: apples (no skins) and applesauce, bananas, grapefruit, lemons, limes, and pears

Vegetables: all cooked vegetables, including potatoes (minimize cooked broccoli, cauliflower, and cabbage as well as potato skins)

Carbohydrates: cornmeal like polenta and corn tortillas, sourdough, white rice and rice products like rice cakes, rice pasta, rice cereals, and rice crackers*

Dairy: cheese, kefir, and yogurt

Fats: avocadoes, extra virgin olive oil, nut butters like peanut butter and almond butter

Protein: fish (no shellfish), soft-cooked eggs (poached, soft-boiled, over-easy), soy/tofu, and whey or rice protein powder

Other: balsamic and apple cider vinegar, black tea, garlic, herb tea, honey, sea salt, and maple syrup

For example, eat sushi; sourdough French toast with maple syrup; a baked potato with steamed veggies, olive oil, sea salt and butter with a piece of baked cod; a peanut butter and natural jelly sandwich on sourdough; fried white rice with "Eden" soy sauce, sautéed vegetables, eggs, and baked tofu; cheese enchiladas; a smoothie with whey protein powder, bananas, rice milk, and frozen strawberries, or one made with protein powder, bananas, and almond butter; plain yogurt with maple syrup; guacamole and corn chips;

salmon, rice, and cooked carrots; polenta with pesto and steamed spinach; cottage cheese and rice cakes; poached eggs, soy sausage and grapefruit... The possibilities with this "limited" list are much greater than it appears.

If you have sensitivity to peanuts, nuts, and/or dairy, do not consume these until this sensitivity has been healed.

* When you initially incorporate these carbohydrates into your diet, replace wheat products like pasta, bread, pizza, and bagels with as many of these carbohydrates instead. Do *not* replace your high protein foods (beef, chicken, pork, turkey) with these, and do not immediately add these into your diet if you have been avoiding carbohydrates altogether.

Chapter Ten

Use The Right Crutch While You Heal

Dietary crutches were discussed in the last chapter. Non-dietary crutches come in the form of vitamins, herbs, and other supplements, exercise, and physical modalities like acupuncture and chiropractic. **This chapter primarily describes how to use supplement crutches effectively so that you can look and feel better while you heal your bowel and body.** For advice on exercise and physical modalities, please consult with a qualified professional in these areas.

Use these non-acidic crutches in place of acidic drugs as much as possible, but do not completely discount the short-term benefits of pharmaceutical drug usage. Also, if surgery will save your life, do not turn it down!

If you don't want to use crutches forever, you have to heal your bowel, as outlined in Chapter 7.

Don't Attempt This Program Without Them

It takes strength to use them

Patiently waiting for your bowel and body to heal is difficult. It takes strength and wisdom to accept that your body needs help while healing. Don't try to be the tough guy who doesn't need help. This serves no purpose other than to increase your chance of failing to achieve your optimum health and weight potential. Clients who use crutches under my guidance are more patient, and therefore more successful, in attaining their ideal health and weight. The crutches also help them understand how their body works, which also increases their chance of success. **Be grateful that crutches exist and take advantage of them.**

You are not a failure if you use these crutches. On the contrary, you are likely to be a failure if you don't.

Are they working for you now?

A large percentage of my clients are using crutches when I first see them. The fact that they have arrived at my office means that the crutches aren't helping, or certainly, not enough. In most cases, they are missing an important crutch, or are simply not taking a strong enough dose of their current crutches. In many cases, I see someone who is taking eight different supplements that all do the same thing, and nothing for the symptom that is most bothersome to them.

If you are currently using crutches, you will still find the following information for using them invaluable in helping you achieve a reduction in your health and weight symptoms while you heal.

Two Reasons a Crutch Won't Work

It's the wrong one

A crutch won't work if you're using the wrong one. If a vitamin B-12 deficiency causes your fatigue and you treat it with adrenal-supporting supplements, for example, your energy will not improve.

It's the right one, just not strong enough

A crutch will not work if it is the right one, but not strong enough. I have clients who have had to take excessively high amounts of a vitamin to feel better. Recently I saw a client who was recommended 3 mg. of melatonin a night for her sleep disturbances. This was not helping. I assessed the condition of her bowel and found it to be very unhealthy. From this I assumed that the crutch was correct, simply not strong enough. I suggested she try 10 mg. at night and sure enough, it worked beautifully. She no longer awoke in the middle of the night, unable to fall asleep. She had more energy during the day, was no longer mentally stressed and frustrated about her sleep problems, and her relationships with her husband and children improved.

Many studies that are done on vitamin usage use very high levels of them over a *short period of time*. There is not much information about the safety of taking vitamins in mega amounts over long periods of time. Personally, I am not willing to experiment with this. Also, my feeling is that if someone needs an excessively high amount of a crutch, or vitamin, it is a reflection that there body is particularly unhealthy, and healing their bowel, in these cases, needs to be especially aggressive. More time and money should be spent doing this. After all, many people won't keep up large amounts of a crutch over time anyway. It is more helpful to focus on large amount of a healing supplement—one that gives cumulative, permanent results and addresses the cause of the problem. In these cases, it is sometimes preferable, and much more effective, for you to utilize medications to look and feel better while you are healing, as these are generally much stronger than natural crutches.

But we keep using them anyway

I have seen many clients over the years that were taking handfuls of supplements, even though they did not see or feel an improvement doing so. Many people seem to think that even if they do not immediately look or feel better, the supplements are still helpful and will keep them healthy. I've seen too many people, including myself, who have taken a lot of supplements as crutches and ended up in a dangerous health situation.

The Right Way to Use a Crutch

In my experience, the number one reason people fail with their crutches is because they are being used incorrectly.

Understand they are just crutches

When I advise crutches to clients, I make it very clear up front that they are treating a symptom and that starting and stopping a crutch is absolutely fine, but that until they heal their bowel and body, their symptoms will only stay improved as long as they keep using them. Used with this understanding, success is dramatically improved.

If they help, don't stop them just because you look or feel better

In other words, because many of you have been led to believe that crutches heal, many of you stop these once you look and/or feel better. Eventually your symptoms and/or weight returns. To succeed with the crutches you are using, you must take them daily, or almost every day. If you stop a crutch and your symptoms or weight problems return, get back on the crutch and realize that you simply have not healed your bowel and body enough to function without it. Your leg isn't fixed yet.

Only use them if they work

If you broke your leg and someone sold you an expensive pair of crutches, you would expect them to immediately be of help to you. If you stood up on the crutches and they were too thin to support you, and they did not help you move around while your leg was broken, you would stop using them.

These crutches should be treated the same way. If you do not look or feel better using them, stop using them. To be fair, give them two weeks to help, as sometimes a crutch is started and the next day you get sick from the flu, for example. Judging the crutches usefulness in this situation would be unfair.

If you don't feel better after taking a crutch for two weeks, don't take it. You may have taken one that is not needed in the first place, a scenario I see all the time. If you don't need it, don't waste your money on it or stress out your body trying to eliminate it. If the crutch doesn't work, it is also possible that you do need it, but your body is too weak for it to help. Sometimes the leg is so badly broken that crutches simply won't help. In this case, it is best to devote your time and money to fixing the weakness in the first place, which means aggressively healing your bowel and body with healing supplements.

Having said that, if you feel "safer" taking a bunch of vitamins, go ahead and do so, as long as it does not distract you from the time and money needed to heal your bowel and body.

Eliminate redundancy

There are many more spaghetti sauces than we really need on the grocery store shelves, and there are many more vitamins than we need as well. Likewise, it is not necessarily beneficial that you buy them all, and it is often not the case that one crutch isn't working while another promises to work because you are missing something.

With the majority of clients that I see, when a crutch isn't working, it is not because it is a bad crutch, or the wrong one; it is simply not strong enough. It is rare that a client understands this, and rather than increasing the dosage, they almost always get sold on the idea that there is a better crutch. This cycle can continue for months, years, or decades! I have seen people go from one good product to another, looking for results, when in reality, they simply needed to increase the dosage of what they were already taking. *The right dose is significantly more important than the brand of crutch that is used.* I have a client who came to me with five products for inflammation, but she suffered from inflammation, still! I had her stop four of them and take only one of them, but at a much higher dosage, and by our next visit two weeks later the inflammation was gone!

259

Often I see a client who has a bunch of different supplements that all do the same thing. Sometimes someone will bring in a bag of thirty products and I will put them in piles according to their function. Often, we end up with a few piles with nine or ten products per pile. The "heal the bowel" pile is always completely lacking or extremely limited.

If you can, find out what all of the stuff that you are taking really does. What symptoms are they helping? Go online or to your health food store and ask for help, if you can't find a nutritionist or other practitioner who can answer this for you. If you have six products that help reduce inflammation, for example, take one at a time. And don't buy more. Most clients have been completely overwhelmed with everything they already have and as a result, they stop all of it. Some people then quit a natural healing approach altogether, while many others just keep buying vitamins, not knowing that they already have ten that do the same thing.

Many people wrongly think that the more different vitamins they take the better. I find this to work to the contrary. Redundancy is usually a deterrent to healing, not a help.

Compare apples to apples and don't stop your current crutches yet

If you are currently using crutches, do not stop them immediately when you start this program. I admire you for wanting to, but this can lead to a wrong misinterpretation of how the healing supplements are working and a greater chance for failure.

For example, if you are using a crutch for your headaches, like chiropractic, and you stop it when you start this program, the headaches will come back, as it takes time to heal and for the headaches to go away naturally. In the very short-term, the increase in headaches can get blamed on the bowel supplements, causing you to stop temporarily or altogether. In truth, the increased headaches occurred because the crutch was stopped too soon.

If you are exercising five days a week, do not stop this yet. Your weight will come back if you stop this before you heal your bowel and body. If you want to reduce this exercise schedule, that is alright, as long as you blame the reduction in your exercise crutch, and not this program, if you gain weight!

If you use a lot of crutches and want to try stopping them, do so one at a time, and do it slowly. If you experience the return of a symptom, restart the crutch, or increase it back to the previous dose, to confirm whether or not you simply yanked it away too soon.

Vitamin crutches are easy to find

Finding a crutch is much easier than you might think. There are natural anti-inflammatory supplements, sleep aids, diuretics, laxatives, anti-oxidants, energy stimulants, and on and on. Companies selling these products will name them so that they are easy to find. For example, a supplement that helps you with your sleep may be called "Sleep Well." Pick a product, any one. If one is on sale, get that one. They are very similar and you are not going to harm yourself. Don't let the large selection scare or confuse you.

I am not going to spend much time here listing all of these and the symptoms they treat because this information is already widely available, and statistics show that many of you are already using them. You can find this information over the Internet, in many books on health at the bookstore, and from the people who work in health food stores. Employees here are trained to sell products to treat your symptoms. They do not have the extensive knowledge needed to understand how to heal your bowel and body and do not expect them to. Use them to help you find crutches; do not rely on them to help you with this program. If you are already seeing an alternative health practitioner, no doubt this person can give you this information as well, in the unlikely case that they haven't already.

Use more if needed

If you start a crutch and do not feel or look better after using it for two weeks, double the dosage for another week and see if that makes a difference. Maybe you have the right crutch, it just isn't strong enough. If you feel or see an improvement within a week of taking a crutch, continue with it if you choose. If you choose to stop it, at the very least, the fact that it helped will provide you with a greater understanding of your condition and ability to change it. If you feel or see no improvement after two weeks, stop it and try to find a better crutch, or put more time and money into the supplements that heal.

I have found all of the crutches that I suggest later on both safe and often effective in dosages higher than the standard recommended amounts. I have had clients take 5,000 mcg of vitamin B-12 a day with no improvements, experience significant improvements in their symptoms after increasing this to 10,000 mcg a day, for example.

My belief is that the greatest danger of taking a high dosage of supplements is not the potential for harm, but the risk of "burn out," and the low likelihood that you will continue with this.

Reduce addictive crutches gradually

Coffee, nicotine, alcohol, recreational drugs, most pharmaceutical drugs, and other addictive substances are crutches that must be reduced gradually. If you try to eliminate these before your body is healthier, you will feel worse. When you feel bad you are likely to fail in healing your bowel and body.

While many programs for addictions rely on a "cold turkey" approach, most people who have followed this advice have failed to remain addiction-free. The approach is wrong, not you.

Many others who have quit cold turkey really have not done this at all. Often an addict will be given pharmaceutical medications, which means that they have simply traded one crutch—the addictive one with a bad name, like cocaine—for another crutch---a pharmaceutical one that is somehow viewed as acceptable. On the other hand, because driving drunk can kill you and other innocent people, it is preferable if you can replace your heavy alcohol crutch with another, like a drug or nicotine, while you heal your bowel and body. I cover addictions in greater detail in *"This Works, Crutches Don't 2."*

As your body becomes healthier, less of a crutch is needed

These crutches are safe to take daily for a very long time. As you heal your bowel and body, however, less of a crutch will be needed to feel and look great, and eventually, none at all. In the meantime, you may use these as long as your bowel is unhealthy and you have health and weight symptoms.

Do not use *Bowel Strength* or acidophilus like a crutch!

Crutches immediately help reduce your health and weight symptoms. They do not heal. On the other hand, *Bowel Strength* and acidophilus heal and cannot immediately reduce your health or weight symptoms. Do not use them as crutches. For example, if you have a headache, increase your intake of calcium, but do not increase your intake of *Bowel Strength* or acidophilus. Not only can these items do nothing to immediately help you feel better, it is possible that once you increase them they will become too strong, making you feel worse, the opposite reaction that you want and need.

Crutches and surgery or blood tests

Some of the crutches listed later on may help your blood tests look better, as blood tests reflect symptoms and crutches treat symptoms. If an abnormal blood test concerns you, especially if it results in pressure to take a drug, I strongly advise you to use these crutches heavily for one week prior to your blood test, including the morning of your test. Also, if your blood tests have always been good, or you haven't had one in a while, take the crutches one week before the tests.

On the contrary, you must stop the *Bowel Strength* or acidophilus for three days prior to your blood tests. This applies to pre-surgery as well.

Read the label carefully!

When you buy a supplement, read the back label carefully for ingredients and serving size. I've had many clients take much too little of one due to a misleading label. For example, sometimes the front label of a calcium supplement will advertise that it contains 1,000 mg of calcium. This is often interpreted to mean that *each capsule* contains 1,000 mg. This is an understanding assumption. On the back label you will see a "serving size." Look at this carefully. It may say a serving size is four capsules, which means that it takes four capsules to give you 1,000 mg, not just one.

Don't stop medication crutches yet

Drugs are more powerful than most natural supplement crutches and must not be discontinued immediately, because you cannot heal your body immediately. The goal is to get off of them eventually.

If you suffer from depression, insomnia, aches and pains, or any other condition that is making life difficult for you—and other approaches to eliminate these symptoms have not worked, including the ideas listed later—consider talking to your doctor and getting a prescription for the next six months or so. While most drugs are acidic, it generally takes a long time of using them before they cause significant harm to your health, and **you will not need them a long time if you heal your bowel and body. You will still be able to heal your bowel and body if you take them. They do not stop the healing process.**

You are not a failure if you use drugs; you are a failure if you feel so uncomfortable that you fail to give yourself the patience needed to heal your body. If you stop a drug you are using and feel horrible, you will be tempted to look for a quick fix, and quick fixes do not heal. You might also be tempted to use a high protein diet crutch to feel better, and this is more harmful to your health than relying on a drug to do this for you. You will also be more likely to need to return to using the drug(s), and this failure can be an emotionally negative experience that you don't need.

As long as you are healing your body you must keep in mind that many medications will become too strong when they are no longer needed, and this can produce symptoms. For example, I have had a number of clients experience jittery, heart-racing symptoms as their thyroid health improved and their thyroid medications became too strong and needed to be stopped.

Find a doctor who is willing to support you in this process and admires your desire to get off of your medications. Let him know that you are healing your body and that you expect them to become too strong at some point. Ask him what symptoms to look for that it is too strong, and ask him how you should handle things if you experience these. Listen to your body. If you are taking medications and you experience any unusual or abnormal symptoms, always contact your doctor to inquire as to whether the medications could be causing them.

When a client goes with the flow and lets the healing process evolve, the elimination of a drug usually occurs naturally and without discomfort. Typically, a client will forget a medication and find that they feel fine off of it.

A lot of strength in a little pill

Drug crutches are much stronger than natural ones and are much easier to take. One tiny little pill may create the same response as twenty supplements. If you cannot take a lot of pills, or won't, the short-term use of a drug may prove valuable to you. If drugs are not strong enough to help, you definitely need to heal your bowel and body. It does not mean there is no hope for you. Your doctor will not risk a lawsuit and prescribe more than is recommended.

Fears of addiction

Many people avoid taking drugs out of concern of the long-term effects of them and of becoming addicted to them. If you heal your bowel, you won't need them in the long-term, and you won't become addicted to them.

Others are afraid of drugs like antibiotics because they have heard that these drugs kill off all of the good bacteria in their bowel. This is completely untrue, and while it is best to use these minimally, do not avoid them when they are necessary—whether they can save your life or you have been very ill for more than a few days and need a quick-fix to get back on your feet and back to work.

You become addicted to drugs when you take them and do nothing to fix the underlying ill health in your body that triggered the symptom or problem in the first place. You become addicted because most of them make your health worse over time. It is as though you have put a tarp over your roof, and the tarp protects your house from getting wet when it rains, but the material of the tarp slowly causes more holes in your roof over time. You will find that if you remove the tarp, your house gets wetter than ever before, and you "need" the tarp to keep your house dry. You are addicted to it. You like a dry house! And the only way this happens is if you continue to use this tarp.

When you heal your bowel and body and fix the holes in your roof, the tarp won't be used long enough to create damage. You will be able to get rid of it--the drug--one day and not "need" it.

My Favorite Crutches

Like all health practitioners, I was taught how to treat symptoms with herbs, vitamins, homeopathic remedies, and other supplement crutches. Early on in my practice I used many of these, along with an emphasis on healing the body by healing the bowel. Due to the lack of powerful bowel-healing products, and experience using them, crutches were needed more.

Now, I put a client's primary focus on aggressively healing their bowel and I recommend a select few, safe and aggressive crutches to help them look and feel better along the way. As mentioned earlier, there are a lot of crutches. The following recommendations are for the ones that I have found to be most helpful. They address 90% of the symptoms that clients present themselves with.

If your bowel is unhealthy these crutches can help you look and feel better. There is no possibility of them making you look or feel worse. Never blame them for these problems. The only exception to this is bentonite, as it is *both a crutch and a healing agent*. If you heal your body too quickly, it can be uncomfortable. Follow the instructions given for its use and you will only look and feel better, not worse.

Make buying and taking the *Bowel Strength* or acidophilus your priority, and then add in a few of the crutches listed below. When I see a client I ask for the top one or two symptoms that bother them the most and try crutches for those first, as I don't want to overwhelm someone with too many pills. For more ideas on which crutches may be best for you, check the list of symptoms and recommended crutches in *This Works Crutches Don't 2*.

The amounts that I have recommended are based on experience and personal knowledge. I have never found them to be unsafe (on the contrary), yet in many cases, they have not been scientifically tested. The recommended amounts are intended for adults, age 18 and older. For children age 5-17, use half the amount, and for children under age 5, contact me for individualized advice, and/or look for *This Works, Crutches Don't For Kids*.

Liquid Bentonite

How it works/symptoms helped

Your bowel is "at the bottom of the pipe" and so bowel symptoms like constipation, poorly formed stools, gas, and bloating, will be the last to become completely eliminated. While you are healing your bowel, bentonite can help reduce (but not completely eliminate) these.

Bentonite is a natural substance that is largely derived from clay that is found in the earth. We have a lot here in Colorado. It helps form up the acids in your bowel that your bowel is not healthy enough to form up on its own. Think of it as an extra trashcan for your front yard to handle the trash that your first trashcan cannot, due to the fact that it has holes in it. Formed acids are not re-absorbed into your blood and body, triggering health and weight problems. Formed acids are eliminated.

Every day that you take bentonite imagine that a man is inside your house with a large shovel, scooping up some trash and throwing it out of your house. Your house will not immediately become clean from this, but over time, the cumulative effect of this will be significant.

As described in Chapter 8, bentonite helps you eliminate acids from your entire body and is healing to every organ. While the full effect of this healing can take some time, a **more immediate response to its use is an improvement in the frequency and form of your stools and less gas and bloating. It is especially helpful for loose stools and diarrhea, but also improves constipation, bloating, gas, stomachaches, yeast infections, and other intestinal discomforts.**

The quicker that you improve the form of your stools, the faster you will eliminate old acids and lose weight, heal your body, eliminate illness, and feel better. I strongly recommend that you use bentontie, if possible.

Having said that, the cause of your diarrhea, gas, bloating, and constipation is an unhealthy bowel, and this takes time to fix. Do not expect bentonite to produce miracles overnight, and keep in mind that, more importantly, every day that you take Bowel Strength or acidophilus, you are addressing the cause of these problems, In other words, even with bentonite, it may take some time before your elimination is ideal. It is very easy to take a laxative and quickly improve the frequency of your stools—which does nothing to eliminate acids or make you healthier; it is not easy to heal your bowel and offset this weakness with bentonite. It is very difficult and complicated to immediately improve the form of your stools, the variable that matters; the variable that helps you eliminate acids and heal your body.

Activated charcoal and Pepto Bismol work the same way as bentonite, but I prefer bentonite as it is stronger and purer. A recent study found that bismuth subsalicylate, as found in Pepto Bismol, inhibits the growth of *H.pylori* and binds or neutralize the toxins of the bacteria, rendering them non-irritating. It decreases intestinal inflammation and increases the activity of intestinal muscles and cells (Stratton CW et al; Bismuth-mediated disruption of the glycocalyx-cell wall of Heliobacter pylori: ultrastructural evidence for a mechanism of action for bismuth salts, *J Antimicrob Chemother* 43(5), 659-66, 1999.)

Disadvantages/misunderstandings of bentonite

To the first-time user, this product can be intimidating due to its thick, beige appearance. It does not taste bad, especially if you dilute it with some water when you take it. The majority of my clients do not have a problem with it.

If you are taking medications, do not take these at the same time you take bentonite, as it absorbs toxins, and drugs are toxic. Wait one hour before or after taking your medications before you take it. Even though I have never personally seen this interfere with someone's medications, it is a standard recommendation that should be followed.

While bentonite can soak up acids in your body—acids that harm you when they are not eliminated—it will not bind to vital nutrients. In fact, because it helps you eliminate acids and because un-eliminated acids are the primary cause of nutritional deficiencies, the use of it will improve, not reduce, your nutritional status. **Bentonite cannot harm you. Un-eliminate acids do.**

If bentonite makes your stools firmer but less frequent, it is not because you are not drinking enough water with it or that it is too strong for you. *If you currently have poorly formed stools and they become less frequent and firmer while taking it, this is a very positive, productive occurrence.* You will look and feel better if you continue with it. The tendency to reduce or stop this product in this case is high, but do not. Please review Chapter 6 for a description of ideal elimination.

On the other hand, if bentonite seems to make your stools looser or infrequent and very hard, stop it. It may be too strong and more than you need. To be sure try it again a few days later to be sure it was the bentonite and not something else that caused this reaction. Unlike other crutches, bentonite is also healing and as a result, taking too much of it can make you feel worse.

In general, as long as you need the Bowel Strength or acidophilus, bentonite should be helpful and comfortable to take. As long as you have holes in your roof, there should be value in using a "mop," like bentonite, to soak up the rain that is getting into your house.

Bentonite works very differently from fiber products and bulking agents. Fiber products do not eliminate acids from your body, bentonite does. If you have had a problem with fiber or bulking agents, it does not mean that you will have a problem with bentonite.

How much do I take?

Bentonite comes in liquid and powdered form. The liquid is preferred by most of my clients. For most of you, 1/4 cup or four tablespoons of bentonite liquid, or 2 teaspoons of bentonite powder, a day will provide noticeable help for your bowels, which will, over time, provide noticeable improvements in your weight and health.

A number of my clients have had great success using much larger quantities but I cannot make that suggestion to you here. If you see some improvements from the amount I suggested but want to go faster, contact me directly so that I can help you do this individually, effectively, and safely.

The brand of bentontie I recommend is by "Yerba Prima" and is called Great Plains Detox.

Bentonite also helps heal your body; it is much more than a crutch. See Chapter 8 for more information on how it helps your body heal and to review the complexities of using this product.

Natural progesterone

How it works/symptoms helped

Natural progesterone is commonly marketed for reducing symptoms of menopause, but this product is not for menopausal women only. Some doctors think progesterone levels can only be low during menopause because they do not understand the role of the bowel in balancing hormones, and that a weak bowel can occur at any age. This weakness may be more noticeable at menopause, but it does not mean that is the only time it occurs and affects you.

I have found natural progesterone very helpful for women of all ages who experience **uncomfortable periods, heavy periods, irregular periods, PMS, pain from fibroids or cysts, nausea, hot flashes, vaginal dryness or pain, miscarriages, unwanted hair, and any other symptoms associated with their hormone levels.** It is also a wonderful crutch for any woman who has or has had **breast or ovarian cancer**, or has a family history of these, as these cancers are largely triggered by the re-absorption of excess estrogen. Progesterone helps balance this excess estrogen, making it less harmful.

Studies show that progesterone improves body temperature. It reduces spasm and relaxes the smooth muscle of the bronchii and is therefore helpful for asthma and sleep apnea. It helps prevent osteoporosis by stimulating osteoblasts, which help bone to heal. It is a neuroprotectant which can be beneficial for multiple sclerosis, memory, brain trauma, epilepsy, and Alzheimer's. It also reduces gallbladder activity, which can have a protective effect on that organ.

Unlike other hormones, there is no chance of water retention and weight gain as a result of using this hormone. If anything, these can be reduced by using natural progesterone.

The use of progesterone for men has not been studied enough, but we do know that is vital for sperm motility and male fertility. Progesterone restores the normal size to the prostate gland. It also reduces the effects of "harmful" testosterone, the kind associated with many cases of prostate cancer. Over the years my client base has consisted of many more women than men, and I have seen tremendous results with natural progesterone with women. Because I do not see nearly as many men, and the ones I do see rarely discuss their sexual and hormonal health with me, I do not have much professional experience using this with men, but I would definitely encourage any man reading this who has these issues to try it.

For more information on natural progesterone read one of the books by Dr. Lee. *"Natural Progesterone"* and *"What Your Doctor May Not Tell You About Menopause"* are especially good. They are available from www.warnerbooks.com.

Disadvantages/misunderstandings of natural progesterone

Failure to understand the complexities of blood pH maintenance and body homeostasis leads to many harmful misinterpretations of how vitamins and other supplements affect your body. Add a little fear to the mixture, and you've got a lot of failures.

Two cases in point: excess calcium in the blood and excess progesterone by the breast cancer site. Excess blood calcium is the result of an overly depleted body that is pulling out the big guns, the calcium in your bones, to keep the un-eliminated acids in your blood from killing you. Likewise, excess progesterone is pulled to the site of excess estrogen to buffer its harmful effects, hence its common presence at the breast cancer site.

If your house is on fire, hopefully firemen will show up to put it out. Progesterone and calcium are the firefighters called on to put out the fires in your body. The firemen do not cause the fire to happen in the first place, anymore than calcium or progesterone cause high blood calcium levels or breast cancer. **Just because you find firemen at a building does not mean they started the fire!**

The fear of using too much progesterone is very common, both as voiced by my clients and from articles on the Internet. Millions of women have been diagnosed with breast and ovarian cancer that were not using these products. Also, I am not aware of any study that has found that giving women extra natural progesterone increases her likelihood of getting or dying from breast or ovarian cancer. I believe every female would be safer if she used progesterone cream while healing her bowel and body. I strongly encourage my female readers to consider this. **My female clients who heal their bowels do not get breast or ovarian cancer.**

Natural progesterone and bio-identical hormones and prescription progesterone are *not* the same.

How much do I take?

Apply ¼ teaspoon of cream to your body two times a day. See the package for further instructions. A standard recommendation is made for you to stop the cream, even if your period is irregular, for seven days from the start of menstrual bleeding. Some of my clients find that they feel bad when they do this and continue with it during their period. While this goes against the conventional recommendation, I have never found it be harmful, on the contrary.

"Emerita" makes the natural progesterone cream that I recommend.

Methyl-vitamin B-12

How it works/symptoms helped

Vitamin B-12 is a necessary nutrient for numerous functions in your body. It is especially helpful in cases of **persistent fatigue, depression, nervous system disorders like multiple sclerosis, nerve pain or discomfort, addictions to alcohol, drugs, exercise, and other items, and sugar cravings. It is also extremely helpful for kids and adults with altered brain chemistry and neurological problems, like autism, ADD, Tourette's, seizures, etc. It is a great crutch to give you the mental strength to handle a long healing process.**

Disadvantages/misunderstandings of vitamin B-12

If you are taking a multivitamin, B-complex, or mega-B vitamins, you will not get nearly enough vitamin B-12. The maximum amount of B-12 in most of these products is 100 or 200 mcg/day. The amount I recommend is 50x stronger than this. High amounts of vitamin B-12 will not cause the other B-vitamins in your body to go out of balance. Finally, all of the B-vitamins, vitamin B-12 included, are water-soluble. This means that if too much is taken it is urinated out of your body, and not stored.

While vitamin B-12 can improve your energy levels it is not a stimulant like caffeine and will not make you jittery or interfere with your sleep. It also cannot give you energy "immediately," so do not use it this way or expect this reaction.

How much do I take?

I recommend 10,000 mcg/day. Use "sublingual, methyl-B-12."

Alkalinizing minerals-- calcium, magnesium, sodium and potassium

How it works/symptoms helped

These alkalinizing minerals are highly abundant in your body, particularly in your bones and intra- and extra-cellular fluids. These minerals buffer un-eliminated acids in your blood. It is like spraying perfume on the trash leaking out of your trashcan. The perfume does not fix the holes that cause it to leak out, nor does it help eliminate the trash, but it sure makes it smell better. These minerals can help you look and feel better because when these un-eliminated acids are buffered, it eliminates your body's symptom and weight reactions to them.

When these acids are buffered you can experience a reduction of many symptoms including, but not limited to: **excess weight, high cholesterol, high blood pressure, reflux, aches and pains, fatigue, high blood sugar, sugar cravings, neurological problems, nighttime urination, asthma, irritability, stress, difficulty falling asleep, and skin problems.**

When I suffered from daily, excruciating neck pain, and getting chiropractic adjustments all the time, I started calcium supplements and went from needing an adjustment daily to just once every two weeks or so.

I read scientific nutritional studies every week. Many of these are done on the benefits of taking extra calcium, magnesium, and potassium. Unfortunately, I never see studies on the benefits of natural sodium, as found in sea salt. All of the studies I do see on sodium test the ill effects of refined, unnatural, harmful salt.

Disadvantages/misunderstandings of calcium, magnesium, sodium, and potassium

Calcium and magnesium

These minerals are recommended for women much more often than for men, even though they are highly beneficial for them as well. Men also have too many un-eliminated acids in their bodies. Generally they have a stronger skeletal system than women and so calcium and magnesium intake is not as important for them as far as reducing their risk of osteoporosis, but all of my male clients benefit—symptom and weight wise—when they add these minerals to their daily intake.

Milk and calcium are not the same. A study finding ill effects of taking calcium did not differentiate between people drinking milk and those taking calcium supplements. Commercials on television say calcium is good and milk contains calcium, and you are meant to conclude, which you do, that it means milk is good for you too. The calcium in milk is not readily available because milk is very difficult to digest. You must be able to digest and absorb calcium for it to be of any value to you.

Taking extra calcium in supplement form does not cause calcium deposits; on the contrary, it can help reduce and eliminate these. The other alkaline minerals have the same benefit. Calcium deposits—like those that contribute to the clogging of your arteries and deposits that turn into gallstones and kidney stones—are the result of un-eliminated acids. When you take in extra calcium and/or other alkaline minerals, you buffer these acids and reduce or prevent these deposits from occurring. Just a few months ago, a medical study was published that reviewed a number of studies looking a the correlation between calcium intake and kidney stone formation and the authors concluded that there was overwhelming evidence that as calcium intake increases, kidney stone formation decreases.

Clients who take the paltry amount of calcium commonly recommended come to me with osteopenia and osteoporosis. Clients who take the larger amounts I recommend see these conditions go away.

Potassium

Twenty years ago there was a popular mulit-level marketing product called "Km." "K" is the symbol for potassium and the "m" represented minerals. It was touted as a cure-all, and I used it for a while. Like all alkalinizing crutches, its value was valid, but its use in healing was not. Like all of these "cures," it eventually disappeared from the marketplace. Nevertheless, potassium is a valuable alkalinizing crutch. I do not make recommendations for it simply because it would take much higher amounts of potassium than the standard amounts recommended for clients to feel better, and my experience is that they prefer larger doses of calcium over potassium; calcium is perceived as a safer crutch.

Sodium/sea salt

Sea salt is alkalinizing and contains a high amount of natural sodium. Regular table salt is acidic and will not alkalinize your blood and is *not* to be used in this recommendation.

Every ¼ teaspoon of sea salt contains 800 mg of sodium. This is roughly equivalent to the amount of sodium that is in an I.V. solution. The sodium in your I.V. while you are hospitalized is enormously beneficial to your immediate well-being. And while all of you would feel and look better if you had access to a daily I.V., you don't. In the 2007 NBA finals one of the star basketball players had the flu on the day of one of the big games, and it was announced that in the morning he was given I.V. fluids, and again at half time. With the flu, he was able to exert himself on the court and perform remarkably well. This would not have been possible without the I.V. How many of you think you could exert yourself on the basketball court for two hours when you've been sick with the flu? Because this player was crucial to the team's success and because winning the finals is worth millions, this player got privileged treatment. Most of us don't have access to this.

In the absence of an I.V., water with added sea salt can be drunk as a preventative or when you are feeling ill, or seem to be retaining too much water. Drink it when you feel achy, headachy, or are particularly tired. Many of your symptoms will improve. How much they improve depends on the relative amount of un-eliminated excess acidity in your body.

If your stools become loose while using this, do not blame the sea salt. It will not make your stools loose. This misunderstanding comes up at times, I believe in response to the use of salts like Epsom salts, as laxatives. Just because a product can increase the frequency of your bowel movements does not mean that it can also make them looser. This is true of sea salt.

If you do not like the taste of sea salt in water, you can add it to beverages or to foods, like soups and sauces. It is just as effective this way.

The benefits of salt have recently been touted for sinus problems in the use of a nasal irrigator called a neti pot. This pot is filled with a salt and baking soda solution. Ages ago we were told to gargle with salt water when we had a sore throat, but this safe and effective recommendation got lost because drugs to eliminate symptoms "are so much easier."

Eating sea salt in the amounts recommended below cannot hurt you. I hear this concern a lot. It is ironic because the average American consumes approximately 3,000 mg of refined, acidic, "hurt you" salt a day, but no one seems to be too concerned about this! This is the salt you should be concerned about. Excess acids can hurt you; neutralizing them with alkaline sea salt will do nothing but help you.

If you are still not convinced that alkalinizing your blood with sea salt will help you look and feel better, try it. For one week, cut out all of the refined salt you eat (avoid going out to eat, and check the labels on the foods you eat!) and eat one teaspoon of sea salt every day. You will be convinced after this.

Baking Soda

Your kidneys make bicarbonates that are used to neutralize acids. Baking soda, or sodium bicarbonate, works the same way. Like sodium and potassium, bicarbonates are electrolytes. I read about using baking soda (and sea salt) to reduce symptoms twenty years ago. It too will immediately reduce your symptoms, but like all of these approaches mentioned here, it is a crutch and needs to be respected as one. It buffers the acids that your unhealthy bowel is not eliminating. It does not heal your bowel, and therefore, like sea salt, it would need to be continued frequently and daily in order to maintain your feelings of improvement. This is neither practical nor appealing.

A client came in with a son who for his ten years of life has been battling asthma and debilitating food allergies. An allergist they had seen had once mentioned the baking soda trick but they had never tried it. It is often difficult to get someone to try something when they are given no explanation for why and how it works. This was true in their case, and since then, they have used it when needed to reduce his asthma symptoms..

How much do I take?

Use calcium citrate or coral calcium only, as these are well absorbed. Many of my clients need to take up to 2500 mg/day to see and feel a difference. If you find a calcium supplement that contains vitamin D, boron, or other minerals or vitamins that is good too. "Now" makes a great line of coral calcium products. "Soloray" makes calcium citrate without added magnesium, and "CitraCal" is a popular calcium citrate product without added magnesium that can be found in discount stores, grocery stores, and drug stores.

Like calcium, the citrate form of magnesium is easiest to absorb. *Do not take a calcium supplement with added magnesium, however, as it is known to have a laxative effect.* If you take magnesium and your stools become loose you may wrongly blame the bowel-healing supplements and fail to heal your bowel and body. Magnesium stearate is a filler used in many supplements and is not to be confused with magnesium citrate. It is listed under "other ingredients." Magnesium stearate does not count as a source of magnesium when looking at these products. (Exception: If you currently take calcium with magnesium, do not change this yet, as you may be relying on the laxative effect of magnesium to prevent constipation, and you could wrongly blame the other products for this constipation if you stop this magnesium crutch right away.)

You do not need magnesium for your body to utilize calcium. By increasing your calcium intake to the amount suggested (2,500 mg/day), you will be reducing the depletion of your magnesium levels because calcium buffers the acids that would otherwise "use up" some magnesium to do so. Also, my clients do not get constipated when they use coral calcium or calcium citrate.

If you purchase coral calcium the label will likely list calcium in the ingredient list twice, once as calcium (from fossilized coral calcium) and then another time as fossilized coral calcium. There will be two different amounts of calcium listed. The one you need to pay attention to is the one listed as "calcium (from fossilized coral calcium), which will have a smaller amount of milligrams of calcium next to it than the other one. If the label says one tablet contains 350 mg of calcium (from fossilized coral calcium) and 1,000 mg of fossilized coral calcium, then each tablet contains 350 mg of calcium (not 1,000).

A common recommendation for potassium intake is 99 mg/day, in the form of potassium chelate, citrate or aspartate. I do not have any professional experience with recommendations above this amount and while the 99mg is helpful, it is not nearly as strong as taking the amount of calcium advised. For this reason, **I strongly recommend that you choose calcium as your alkalinizing mineral crutch.**

Sea salt and baking soda can be used at the same dose, which is one teaspoon in approximately one cup of water. I have had clients respond well to more, but few will maintain this for very long. These two products are very inexpensive, but if you can't stomach their taste, use calcium instead.

I cannot guarantee that these recommended dosages will neutralize 100% of your un-eliminated acids. The more you have, the less benefit you will see from these. If calcium doesn't help you, consider that your bowel is very unhealthy and there are too many un-eliminated acids for it to buffer. This should be your signal that your bowel is very dangerously weak and your focus should be placed on aggressively healing it. After some time of doing so, these recommendations for calcium will be much more helpful.

Where do I purchase these?

All of these supplement crutches can be found at a health food store or online. Bentonite can generally be found in health food stores, near the fiber products, but sometimes it is hard to find. Many of my clients purchase bentonite online and have had a great experience doing so, although occasionally the bottles break during shipping, so if it has been more than five days since you placed your order, call and inquire about it. I have no affiliation with the following companies and make no money from your purchases from them, but suggest two, www.iherb.com, and www.herbspro.com (866-915-5300). If you have further questions or concerns about these products, please, contact the company that sells them.

Don't worry about the company selling the product. It is more important to use the right crutch, in the right way, at the right dose, than the actual brand name. Companies want you to believe that their product is special and unique, because that is what they rely upon to get you to buy theirs and not someone else's supplements, but in reality, the brand name is mostly irrelevant to your success with it.

I don't carry most of these crutches because you can get high quality ones at a price less than I can charge, and I'm all for you saving money.

Can too much be harmful?

Not only is one unlikely to take a very large amount of supplements every day for the rest of their life, the effects of this on the body are not well known. Studies are very expensive and largely done if the group sponsoring the study seeks to profit from it. Doing a long-term study that measures the effects of massive supplementation on the body has tremendous value, but it is simply not done.

Is it safe to use high amounts long-term? Who knows? I believe it is significantly safer than using drugs long-term, or eating a long-term high protein diet. I consider the amounts that I have listed in the following sections to be extremely safe.

I would feel much safer taking a very high dose of calcium, for example, than using a prescription anti-inflammatory to ease my pains, if I had them. If 1,200 mg of calcium does not eliminate your headaches but 3,000 mg does, but gosh, that is more than "they" recommend, do you think it is safer to take a drug to eliminate your pain, or to take the higher amount of calcium? I would definitely say the calcium is significantly safer, but that is simply based on my knowledge and experience, as it has not been scientifically proven.

The environment of fear about using supplements has been very misplaced. Much more harm and death is attributable to the use of medications, drugs, and the consumption of salt, animal products like chicken and beef, alcohol, and sugar, but the collective fear around the use of these substances is, wrongly, much lower.

In my experience, it is *much* more harmful to take too few of these crutches than to take a large amount of them.

Watch Out For These Crutches

Some commonly recommended crutches need to be used with caution. They are: vitamin C; magnesium, senna, aloe, cascara, rhubarb, and any other laxative-type products that stimulate your bowels to move; any herbs or vitamins that stimulate uterine contractions, if pregnant; and any herbs or vitamins that stimulate your heart if you have a weak one. Also, vitamin A, D, and E are fat-soluble and if more is taken than needed, these can become stored in your body at dangerous levels. Excess amounts are not merely urinated from your system as many other nutrients are. In my practice, I do not routinely make recommendations for any of these, except where a modest amount of vitamin D is included in some calcium supplements. (I know that vitamin D is currently the "magic cure all," but I would be careful about jumping on this bandwagon is I were you.)

Vitamin C

Many of you have been told only one side of the story about vitamin C, and many of you have been sold on it as a cure-all, powerful protector of your health. It is not that simple. I have helped many clients who arrived at my door with a long history of taking this vitamin regain their health.

I am a fan of vitamin C, but it must be used carefully and individually. This is not happening. Many years ago it was common knowledge that the dosage of vitamin C that you took should be lowered if it caused your bowels to become loose. I find this necessary knowledge to be almost nonexistent now. It is imperative that you follow it, however. If you get loose stools when you take vitamin C it means that it is too strong for your body and can cause *more* problems, not less, if you continue with it. **You are not eliminating health-reducing and weight-causing acids when your stools are loose!** Many of my clients have loose stools when they come to see me, and if you do too, you should not be taking large amounts of vitamin C, which is any amount over 500 mg/day. The other day I advised a client who came to me with uncomfortable bloating to stop the 1,000 mg of vitamin C a day that she was taking and she experienced an immediate improvement in her bloating.

When I was ill I took five to ten grams, or 5000-10,000 mg, a day for several years. At one point I even had ten grams intravenously dripped into my veins. I never once got loose bowels because of it. On the contrary, I always suffered from constipation. In my case the vitamin C was a helpful supplement. As I healed my body this became too strong and I eventually stopped it.

Vitamin C is unlike many other vitamins as it is cleansing. It can move acids from your blood and lymphatic system into your bowel. It moves trash into your trashcan. Too much acidity in your lymphatic system makes you more susceptible to viral infections like colds—hence its notorious use for these—but when you shove this acidity into your bowel and your bowel is weak and cannot handle it, you are now more susceptible to a bacterial infection. I have seen this occur time and again. I have had many clients take vitamin C when they had a cold—without my recommendation—only to call me a week or more later to tell me that they were still very sick and had to eventually take an antibiotic to get better. Trading your viral infection for a bacterial one is not productive or desirable.

I have advised many clients to stop their vitamin C, even though this has evoked in many of them a fear of getting sick. Rachel Johnson, Ph.D. cited a review of 29 studies involving more than 11,000 participants that found that Vitamin C failed to reduce the incidence of colds. I have yet to find a study that measures the effect of taking vitamin C and the greater incidence of bacterial infections because of it, but it deserves one, and I am confident a correlation would be found. In the meantime, the safest and most effective way to reduce viral infections like colds is to heal your bowel, as a healthy bowel prevents the re-absorption of acids into your lymphatic system that causes it to be weak and vulnerable to them.

It is safer and more effective to take 50 mg of chelated zinc to reduce your symptoms of a cold.

Aloe, senna, cascara sagrada, and rhubarb, and other laxatives

Many bowel and weight loss products contain these ingredients, which act like a laxative, stimulating your bowel to contract more intensely. This produces more frequent bowel movements, which can result in the loss of water through loose stools and dehydration, which can be dangerous. If you take one of these and your bowels become loose and more than one time a day, your must stop it.

Products that contain laxatives are very popular because these ingredients immediately increase bowel movements, and everyone loves what they (wrongly) perceive as a quick fix of their bowels! It sells a lot of products. Just the other day a client came in with a new product I had never seen that is used for weight loss and constipation. Sure enough, it contains a laxative called Malva leaves. I had to look this up online as I had never heard of it before. The point is, there are many herbs that have a laxative effect that should be used very carefully. I cannot list all of them here, so before you are tempted to take a "magic product," do some research first.

Some clients need these supplements as a mental crutch, as their constipation can cause them a lot of mental anguish. If this is you, it would be better to use bentonite. If you still don't understand how and why bentonite helps with constipation, go back and review the concepts in Chapter 6 of how stools are formed. Bentonite is healing; **laxatives do nothing to make you or your bowel healthier.**

Vitamins, herbs, and pregnancy

If you are pregnant or nursing, consult with your physician before taking any supplements. Most specifically, you do not want to take herbs like black and blue cohosh that can stimulate uterine contractions. None of the products that I recommend contain these. You also should not take supplements that have the potential to cause problems if they are too strong, like *Bowel Strength*, and acidophilus (and vitamin C). While I have had all of my pregnant clients use these supplements successfully and in a way that offered great help, I would and could not offer that advice without individually consulting with you.

In Summary

Start *Bowel Strength* or acidophilus. Take as much as you can tolerate and per the instructions given in Chapter 7. Plan on taking these for a minimum of one year, or longer, depending on the health of your bowel when you start this program and your health goals.

While you are healing your bowel with these products, use bentonite, calcium, vitamin B-12, and progesterone cream, if appropriate. Use these crutches to reduce your health and weight symptoms quickly and plan on using them, at least to some degree, until your bowel and body have been healed.

While you are healing your bowel and body, replace as many highly acidic, hard to digest foods with more alkalinizing, easier to digest ones, as described in Chapter 9.

A complex process that is more than worth it

All of the products mentioned in this book do not simply heal your bowel and body and eliminate your symptoms, illness, addictions, and weight struggles. *They can only do this if they are used correctly. Take the time to review the information and instructions in this book so that they are.*

The fine line between success and failure in achieving your health and weight potential in this program depends upon patience and persistence.

If you are not getting the results that you should, this program is not failing you. You are following it incorrectly. If this is you, contact me at www.ThisWorksCrutchesDont.com **to schedule an appointment so I can help you attain the success that is possible with this program, and that you deserve.**

Quick Order Form

Book orders:

To order additional copies of this book, contact Author House at 1-888-280-7715 or www.authorhouse.com. Click on the link up top for "Book Store" and follow the instructions. You can also request a copy from your local bookstore.

***Bowel Strength* can be ordered through me in either of the following ways:**

Email orders (for speediest delivery): To pay with PayPal, go to the supplement order page of my website www.ThisWorksCrutchesDont.com.

Fax orders: 303-449-5738. Please fill out this form and include your credit card information.

Telephone orders: Call 303-440-3559. Have your credit card ready.

Postal orders: Donna Pessin, 2885 Aurora Ave. Suite 19, Boulder, CO 80303, USA.

Please send me _____bottles of *Bowel Strength*. I have included $30 plus $2 shipping and handling for each bottle purchased.

Total amount to be billed/enclosed: $_____

_____I have enclosed a check, payable to Donna Pessin _____Please bill my credit card:

Visa/Mastercard_____Number_____

Name on the card_____

Exp. Date_____

Please send me FREE information on:

_____Consulting   _____Speaking/seminars   _____Other books

Name:_____

Address:_____

City:_____State:_____
Zip:_____

Telephone:_____

Email address:_____

If Ship To address is different please provide that below:

Name:_____

Address:_____

City:_____State:_____
Zip:_____

All orders will be shipped as soon as possible.